LIVING
BY DESIGN

Discovering the Spirit,
Soul, and Body Connection

RAY D. STRAND, M.D. AND BILL EWING
WITH TODD HILLARD

Every effort has been made to make this book as accurate as possible. The purpose of this book is to educate. It is the review of Scripture and scientific evidence, which is presented for information purposes. No individual should use the information in this book for self-diagnosis, treatment, or justification in accepting or declining any medical therapy for any health problems or diseases. Any application of the advice herein is at the reader's own discretion and risk. Therefore, any individual with a specific health problem or who is taking medications must first seek advice from their personal physician or health care provider before starting a nutritional program. The authors and Real Life Press shall have neither liability nor responsibility to any person or entity with respect to loss, damage, or injury caused or alleged to be caused directly or indirectly by the information contained in this book. We assume no responsibility for errors, inaccuracies, omissions, or any inconsistency herein. Any slights of people, places, or organizations are unintentional.

Printed in the United States of America

First printing 2006

ISBN 0-9747308-1-5

Cover Illustration by Adriane Wright, Salt Lake City, Utah.
Jacket design and typesetting was provided by tmdesigns in Salt Lake City, Utah.
www.tmdesigns-slc.com

ATTENTION MEDICAL FACILITIES, CORPORATIONS, UNIVERSITIES, COLLEGES, AND PROFESSIONAL ORGANIZATIONS: Quantity discounts are available on bulk purchases of this book for educational purposes. Special books or book excerpts can also be created to fit specific needs. For information, please contact Real Life Press, P.O. Box 9226, Rapid City, SD 57709.

This book is dedicated to our children,

their spouses,

and the generations to come.

Jesse and Janie

Nic, Sherri, and Cali

Kyle

Donny and Jessica

Nick and Sara

Sarah and Ryan

Acknowledgements

There are many individuals we wish to thank who have contributed to the production of this book. First, and most of all, we want to thank Todd Hillard for his wonderful collaboration on this project. Without his personal involvement and efforts in this project, this book would not have been completed. He is a wonderful writer who was able to take our message and give it that special touch. He became as deeply involved as we were in the message of this book. Thank you Todd for the wonderful time we have been able to share working together on this book.

We would also like to thank all of the staff at Christian Life Ministries who have strongly supported us during this project. Their guidance and constructive criticism have helped this message crystallize in our hearts and minds. We especially want to thank Pat Karn and Dave Shupe whose direction and input was very important in the creation of this book.

A special thanks needs to be extended to our editors and proof readers Sharon Smith, Daisy Martin, and Bob and Helen Folsland. They poured over our manuscript and gave it that finished touch. Also, we want to extend special thanks Dr. Terry Altstiel who helped us create the final direction and message for the book.

In a project that involves so much time and effort, we want to take the time to share our gratitude to our wives Nancy and Liz. Without their support and help a project like this would never have come to fruition. We especially want to thank Nancy who spent a considerable amount of time pouring over the manuscript and helping us with our scripture verses and quotes. Her insight and tremendous literary talent has been so helpful during this entire project.

The personal insights into God's word that are shared in this book are the result of a lifetime of our personal journey of knowing more and more about Him. We hope and pray that this book touches your life as much as it has touched ours.

Table of Contents

Introduction

Now may the God of peace Himself sanctify you entirely;

and may your spirit and soul and body be preserved

complete,

without blame at the coming of our Lord Jesus Christ.

Faithful is He who called you, and He also will bring it to

pass.

1 THESSALONIANS 5:23-24

When the apostle Paul wrote these words nearly 2,000 years ago, he wrote to those who were living in circumstances not unlike our own. The "modern" world of Thessalonica in the year 55 AD was filled with uncertainty, difficulty, and ungodliness. Those who called themselves "believers" were few and faced many difficult issues. These included division in the church, broken family relationships, fear of death, and the deceptive messages of those people who sought to destroy those of faith.

Some things never seem to change, do they? What the Thessalonians faced, we face. The trials that they shared, we share. Stress, illness, conflict, and the pending and certainty of death have been a part of the human experience since just after the dawn of creation leaving us in a wake of tension and illness.

What is one to do about it?

When I went to medical school at the University of Colorado, I trained to be a member of the most advanced medical community on the planet. When I received my M. D. degree and began to practice, I did so with great expectations, looking forward to a career that would help others in tangible ways. But I immediately found out that I could accomplish only so much. Even in the United States, the inadequacies of medical science are vast. Even when we did our best, illness and death eventually prevailed, taking not only health and life but also hope.

This all changed when two men came into my life. First and foremost was Jesus Christ. He started a transformation that changed everything I thought I was and everything I thought I was to do. It's a transformation that continues day after day as I learn to walk in His Spirit moment-by-moment.

The second person to change my life was a man named Bill Ewing. The son of one of the nurses in my office, I had followed his professional baseball career and began an endearing friendship with him when he returned to our hometown to begin a biblical counseling center called "Christian Life Ministries." From the beginning, Bill has been an integral part of my spiritual growth. In many ways he was, and is, my spiritual leader. Over the decades, we've spent a lot of time together, treating and ministering to those who were not only sick, but also those who were sick of life.

As we began to refer clients to each other, we began to see a common denominator. This thread that wove itself through the minds, emotions, and bodies of nearly everyone who came through either of our offices was stress. Stress was robbing people of joy, distracting them from their relationship with God, and destroying their health. Christians seemed to hold no advantage in their battles against anxiety and illness. Regardless of their religion, their souls and flesh were ravaged by stress stealing their peace and attacking their bodies.

When we looked at the lives of our patients and clients (and when we took an honest look at our own lives), it was clear that something was amiss. Something was fundamentally wrong in how life was being lived. What was it?

In Paul's message to the Thessalonians, the central issues behind the core problem was obvious: "The God of peace" desired that the "spirit and soul and body be preserved complete..." and it was promised that, "Faithful is He who called you, and He also will bring it to pass." Fueled by our own frustrations, and confirmed by numerous passages in the living Word of God, Bill and I came to two realizations: First, we were convinced that we needed to be ministering to the *whole* person, not just parts. According to Scripture, the *complete* person encompasses the spirit, the soul, and the body. Scripture clearly instructs us to make a distinction between these three elements of our being—elements that make a human complete and make us completely human—for each serves an indispensable role for us during the short years we have on this earth. Yet at the same time, the spirit, soul, and body are inseparably linked, displaying a unity and an intermingling that makes us one complete person.

Our first realization was that people focused on one area at the expense of the other two. Christians normally show great concern for spiritual growth, yet display tremendous neglect for the physical body. Others are so consumed with physical appearance and health that they have little passion or focus left for eternal purposes. Some are so concerned with intellectual religious knowledge, that they have never personally found spiritual rebirth at all. The fact is that when one element is neglected, all are affected. When the soul is filled with conflict and tension, the stress radiates into every part of the body, often incapacitating us for God's work and worship. Certainly this was the case when we looked at our Christian clients. Stress, anxiety, panic attacks, and depression have deprived the true believer in Christ and taken away their peace. Oftentimes physical issues interfered with mental ones, and these mental issues affected emotional ones, and so on.

Our second realization was that the Christian life was not at all what it appeared to be. We learned (often the hard way) that God's way is counter-intuitive, radically unreligious, and more different and intriguing than anything we could imagine or think. We began to live out the mystery and simplicity of the Gospel, having discovered the key principles of faith—principles that are taught by only a few, understood by even fewer, and applied by only a handful. For two millennia, these truths have been obvious in Scripture, available to any who lets the Word of God speak for itself. Yet they have been undiscovered by many of those who share the faith.

Between these two realizations, we've found that there are a handful of essential concepts that are indispensable for daily living. They reflect the reality that life, as we know it, is the result of the planned actions and intentions of a personal God—an all knowing and loving God who designed the spirit, soul, and body to function in certain ways, even in a fallen, painful world. It's a design of hope, answering the core questions of our existence:

- How victory and peace come not from what you do, but from what God has done.
- How you can be "reconciled" to God, others, and self.
- Why the "mind" and "will" are central to all life change.
- How your life is now Christ's life—and how resting in that fact

is the fundamental key that unlocks every mystery and solves every riddle.
- How your body was designed to work, and how to optimize it through exercise and nutrition.
- What to do when you face struggles through illness and difficulty.
- How illness and death are to be viewed from an eternal perspective.

As these principles became clearer and clearer, our passion grew to create a book that integrates the infallible principles of the Bible with the best of medical science in a way that illuminates God's designed function for the spirit, soul, and body. In the pages ahead, we are offering a complete, and for many a *completely new,* paradigm for life. You'll find a mixture of cutting-edge health research presented in the broader context of scriptural truth. The work of Bill Ewing permeates every page with biblical concepts that touch the soul where it needs it the most, and offers a spiritual perspective on an extremely practical level. As you begin to understand how God designed you, you'll see that your spirit, soul, and body *can* work together in union as God intended. And when it does, peace and vision prevail...even in the midst of difficult circumstance ... even in the face of physical death.

What God has revealed will push your faith to the edge of its boundaries ... and beyond, pointing you to freedom and maturity. As you immerse yourself into a deeper relationship with the Creator, you'll discover that following His design leads to an existence that is passionate, purposeful, and empowered by His very presence in your heart.

And that's important, for one day, this earth and all of God's material creation will pass away. It's only a matter of time. The heavens will pass away, the earth will pass away, and our bodies will return to the dust from which they came. Someday, the world and the universe as we know it will no longer exist. And someday, even time as we know it will be absorbed into the eternal presence of our loving Creator.

That's part of the design too. From the ashes of this certain reality comes an urgent and crucial imperative: *Live life by design.* It's a design that transcends earthly pain and death, igniting a vision for eternity; allowing us to see each present moment with clarity and direction.

May God give us the courage and wisdom to live out our remaining days, be they many or be they few, in accordance with His divine design.

–Ray Strand, M.D., 2006

The Design

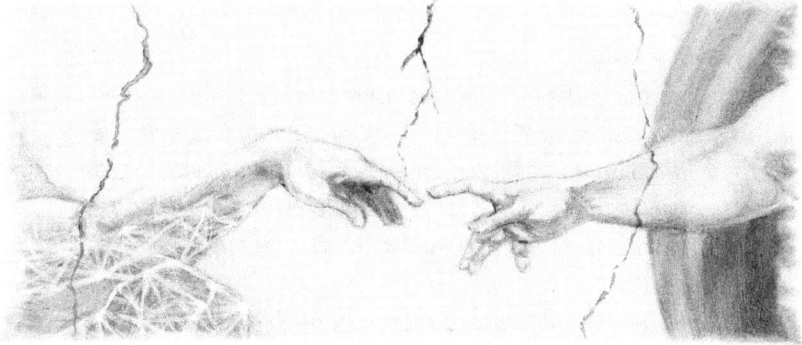

Living by Design begins with a foundational understanding of how our Creator has designed us. As a counselor and a physician respectively, Bill and I have spent decades contemplating the human design from differing, but overlapping, disciplines. I, from the perspective of a physician, have literally cut deep into the human body, exploring its intricacies. Bill, from the perspective of a counselor, has seen the human soul at its best and at its worst. Together, as men of faith, we have shared great interest in the workings of the human spirit—and it has left us in wonder and amazement.

Something that intrigued us is the "comprehensive integration" of God's design. By that we mean that every part of our being is connected to and influenced by every other part. The soul affects the body; the body affects the soul; and the spirit serves as the unifying core—around which all other aspects of our being revolves. As our friendship and respect for each other has grown, a steady path of patients and clients has flowed between our two offices. Bill recognizes that physical problems within the body are sometimes responsible for a client's emotional struggles and regularly refers people to me for medical help. I on the other hand have been involved in treating many diseases and illnesses which are, in part, a result of wrong thinking and spiritual confusion. In those cases, I often need to send my patients to Bill for counseling.

Through it all we both see the continued ravages of stress. A consequence of living in a sin-laced and "fallen" world, stress sends shockwaves into every aspect of our being. Recognizing stress is the first step, for once this foe is revealed, God's truth can be used to bring us to victory over it.

Our Creator God,

As we now begin the incredible journey into life as You designed it, we ask that You would draw us to Yourself in both wisdom and humility. Teach us and show us truth, both through the timeless Scriptures and the ever-growing knowledge of science. Reveal to us the principles and the information that lie at the foundation of our Christian existence, that we might enjoy this life to its fullest measure.

As we probe the magnificent blueprint of Your original design, draw us to our knees in humility. Let us come and bow down and worship, kneeling before You as our Lord and as our Maker. For You are our God, and we are the work of Your hands. Anything right in who we are is from You and You alone. To You and You alone be the praise.

Amen

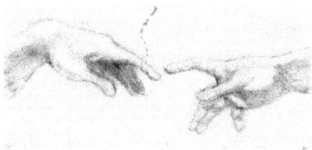

CHAPTER 1

Spirit, Soul, and Body

In the beginning God created...

GENESIS 1:1

Men go abroad to wonder at the height of mountains,
at the huge waves of the sea, at the long courses of the rivers,
at the vast compass of the ocean, at the circular motion
of the stars; and they pass by themselves without wondering."

SAINT AUGUSTINE

In the beginning, there was nothing—a nothing unlike anything that can be imagined: A darkness with no contrasting light; an emptiness with no boundaries; distance without anything to measure it. It was a nothing before the first atom, before the first molecule, before the first photon of energy. It was the time before there was time—and the nothingness reached back into eternity past.

3

But in the midst of the nothing there was an intention, an objective, an idea; for in the midst was One who encompassed the nothingness. His love and truth permeated the void... and then He chose to transcend it.

In the beginning, the voice of God spoke into the nothing. From the reverberation of His heart a plan exploded that was so grand it absorbed everything that was not. As time and space emerged from the nothing, God's hand orchestrated a symphony that molded and shaped a universe. As He spoke, His voice spread through His love and revealed a design that reaches from the minuteness of each single electron to the expanse of the farthest galaxy. Yet in all its brilliance, it was only a dim reflection of the character of the Hand that had made it.

So in the beginning, He created a home. A home filled with light and moisture and rich soils that would be home to the greatest of all His creations. From His touch upon the dirt and the infiltrating breath of His Spirit He formed a man... and from the man, a woman. In their perfect humanity, in the perfect place, they reflected His image, walking in communion with the One who made them.

That was the design. And it was good. In fact, it was very good.

Certainly, things have changed from those days of perfection. Today we see the Designer through distorted eyes, and live a life that is a decaying remnant of the original design. Still, everywhere we turn we are reminded that there is a Designer. Many of us who believe that He exists have never considered the implications of His creation... and then there are those who deny both a design and the Designer entirely.

During my years as a pre-med student, I took many courses in biology and other sciences. Without exception, my professors presented evolution as though it were an established scientific fact, and none of us thought to challenge it. One of my biology professors told the class that human evolution began with the "fact" that an amoeba crawled out of the water and on to the sand. Then a wart became a leg and a freckle evolved into an eye. Eventually, man just evolved.

When I was studying anatomy and physiology in my first year of medical school, I thought about what my professor had told me a couple of years earlier about how he believed that the eye evolved from a freckle on that amoeba. But as I looked at the basic anatomy of the eye and physiology of the eye, something came alive in my soul, and I became enthralled with the complexity and beauty of how the eye actually works:

The act of seeing begins with the capture of images focused by the cornea and lens upon a light-sensitive membrane in the back of the eye, called the retina. Light is absorbed by photopigment in two classes of receptors: rods and cones. There are approximately 100 million rods and 5 million cones in the human retina. Rods operate under dim illumination and cones operate under daylight conditions and are specialized for color perception and high spatial resolution. Photoreceptors are sensitive to light and when stimulated pass this information along the optic nerves to the visual centers within the brain through millions of ganglion cells in each retina.

The majority of ganglion fibers connect to the primary visual cortex of the brain. This massive and continuous sensory input of light from the eye is interpreted by the brain into pure vision. The human eye and brain are able to differentiate over a million different colors and bring it all into a perfectly focused and moving picture of the world around us.

As I studied the eye in more and more detail, I just had to sit back and marvel at how intricate and miraculous the eye was, along with the gift of sight. I did not have a personal relationship with the Lord at that time, however, I was truly in awe of what I was seeing. *The eye is the result of an accident and had evolved from a freckle on an amoeba?* I just shook my head and thought to myself, *I just don't have that much faith.* The eye and the entire body for that matter *had* to be the result of intelligent design. There was no other explanation. At that moment, in that class, I began to see things differently. I glanced down at the ink pen I was holding. *Could some ink, plastic, and metal just sit around for millions and millions of years and accidentally form into the pen I was holding?* It was impossible. *Someone had to make it.*

Romans 1:20 says, "For since the creation of the world His invisible attributes, His eternal power and divine nature, have been clearly seen, being understood through what has been made, so that they are without excuse." Since that day in class, I have found myself looking with awe and amazement at the creation that is all around me. The next time you take a walk outdoors away from the city take a close look at what has been created around you. Is this all an accident or the result of a big bang or perhaps the result of an intelligent design from an all-knowing and all-loving Creator? Then stop and take a look at yourself. The complexity of our mere existence is phenomenal. Just the *thought* of walking sets off a complex neuromuscular response that allows you to move throughout this wonderful creation. Your "gaze" at the trees, birds, animals, and sky is actually a complex and intricate focus of light images that the brain is able to interpret into that wonderful gift of sight. Marvel at the many different colors you are able to see in three dimensions. Touch the soft petal of a flower and smell its beautiful aroma. You can't help but reflect on God's invisible attributes, His eternal power, and His divine nature, which are *clearly* seen by what He has created.

Of all things found in nature, however, the crowning jewel of all He made is the human being. Mankind is truly the most astounding creation of all! And it is by design, and not by chance, that we have been brought here.

Spirit, Soul, and Body

To better understand how God has created us, we need to first define and break down the *parts* that together make us *whole* and complete.

The *Human* Body

The human body is a majestic creation, remarkable in its intricate complexity. The wonder of sight is only one of thousands of examples of His craftsmanship. The body allows us to relate to the world through our senses and to function in our environment. When we consider the body's ability to absorb massive amounts of sensory input and process all of this into our memory, we can't help but marvel at its design. However, the human body, by itself, is merely an "earth suit" that houses our soul and the human spirit. It is strictly designed to live on this earth, and in very limited places. If you place the body one foot below the water or on the highest mountain, it is able to survive for only a few minutes or just a few days. However, it is perfectly designed to exist in our normal atmosphere and climate (with proper clothing, shelter, and protection).

Our lungs, for example, are able to provide the proper amount of oxygen from the air around us. This oxygen is picked up by the red blood cells as they pass through our lungs and they transport it to every cell in our body via the cardiovascular system. We are able to digest and absorb our food through the gastrointestinal tract, which provides us the minerals, antioxidants, vitamins, and fuel that the body requires to survive on this planet. Every cell in our body is able to utilize oxygen, micronutrients, and macronutrients, which then allows the body to function as God intended.

Consider the brain. It is able to gather tremendous amounts of information from our senses and process it quickly. It is also the control center for every system in the body. Messages and control signals generated in the brain are sent to every organ in the body .These signals can be generated by our conscious mind but many of these signals are generated by the unconscious mind. Memories from our early childhood to the present time have all been stored in the memory banks of our brain. Isn't it amazing that you still can even recall things that happened to you when you were four or five years old? The brain and its function have largely remained a mystery to researchers. How can something this small accomplish so much?

I have spent my entire adult life studying and learning how to help my patients protect and even regain their health. The intricate and complex systems that are required to allow us to survive on this planet are unbelievable. The immune, excretory, musculoskeletal, digestive, neurological, respiratory, and cardiovascular systems are just some of the amazing aspects of the human body.

The human body, however, pales in comparison to the magnificence of our souls.

The Human Soul

The soul stands between the spirit with its openness
to the spiritual world, and the body, which is open
to the physical world... having the power of choice
as to which shall control the entire man.

JESSIE PENN-LEWIS

The human soul gives us *conscious awareness* of what is happening around us, *feelings* to show us what is happening within us, and a *will* to make decisions based on what we conclude is "true" about what is best for us. Emerging from the soul are the roots of our "personality" and "self-awareness." The soul gives us the capacity to think—even to think about our thoughts—and contemplate our existence and being.

As a counselor, Bill has spent most of his days ministering to people on a soul level. Even after twenty-five years and thousands of clients, the capability and complexity of the human soul still astounds him. I've always been amazed by the design of the human soul. Our "minds" gather, process, and evaluate huge amounts of data while formulating complex views of the world, others, God, and ourselves. The "will" is the great command and control center of the soul—where all of our conscious decisions are made. The will makes "the call" after considering input from the mind, the spirit, and the emotions.

"Emotions" are *reactions* to what is going on in the mind and body; acting like a thermometer that reveals our soul's inner condition. For example, just a moment ago, as I was sitting here typing, I noticed a black creature moving across the table. A quick jolt of fear startled me and I jumped back. Rerunning this in slow motion, what just happened? My eyes sent the image of the black creature to my brain where my mind gathered the information and quickly processed the data. That data was compared with past knowledge stored in my memory: (spider, black round-shaped back, red hourglass underside,) and concludes: black widow, poisonous, deathly dangerous! My mind, in an instant, sent this information to my emotions. The alarm and fear triggered my will to jump back or attack. In this instance my emotions responded only semi accurately (it was a beetle, not a black widow), revealing the huge problem with emotions: They don't have "intelligence." They can only *respond,* and often do so in error.

Suppose you awake in the morning to a terrible snowstorm producing zero visibility. You know that your son traveled to a distant city last evening. You are suddenly filled with panic and anxiety and picture him stranded on the side of the road with a stalled car, temperatures below freezing, and no coat. While throwing on your coat to go look for him the telephone rings. It is your son. Wiser than you gave him credit for; he hasn't left his friend's house!

Emotions were not designed to be our guide, but rather our gauges. Therefore, emotions should *not* be used to guide our life. They must be interpreted alongside of truth, and then wisdom and our will should be used to act accordingly. Sometimes our choices will be in accordance with our emotions if the emotions align with truth. Sometimes we must act contrary to our emotions when they do not align with truth.

Understandably, emotions have unusual power to affect the health of our bodies. *A single emotion sets in motion a complex series of chemical reactions that impact every cell in the body.* When we train ourselves to use our minds, rather than emotions, we can make choices based on what the Word says is spiritually true—and every aspect of our soul and body benefit.

The Human Spirit

As humans, we share some common things with the other living members of creation. Plants, for example, have bodies. Look at any vegetable or tree or flower and you will quickly see that the body of a plant provides the nourishment (roots), structure (trunk or stem), and the manufacturing source for energy and growth (leaves). Animals possess bodies too, but they also have a soul with the ability to think, feel, and act. They have also been given amazing instincts, which allow them to survive and thrive. However, God created us differently. *Rather than being created to live primarily by instinct, we were created not only with a body and a soul but also with a human spirit that was designed to house His Spirit.* The spirit is the *real you*. It is from our spirit—inhabited by God's Spirit—that we were designed to live. This is living by design ...God's design.

Perhaps nothing is as intriguing or elusive as the human spirit. It is a mystery in so many ways, yet God designed the human spirit as the means to guide and control our soul via His indwelling Spirit. In the design of the human spirit, we see a reflection of the heart of God, for He designed it as a vessel in which a human and God could—and should—live together, united in perfect intimacy. In this way, the human spirit can serve as the bridge between man and God. It's the place where the things of the body and soul mesh, with familiarity and confidence; the place where all of our deepest needs for communion and love are fulfilled.

For a period of time, at the dawn of human existence, it was so: a man and a woman, walking moment-by-moment with the Father in a garden that knew only life. They had unblemished bodies with which to love each other and to soak in the beauty and provision of Eden. Their souls knew nothing but truth. Their minds, wills, and emotions worked in harmony, in innocence, and in freedom. The balance of life was so exceptional that Adam and Eve were "naked and were not ashamed" (Genesis 2:25). They walked without a hint of guilt, threat, or fear of punishment—and therefore without any of the stress we know in this present day.

In the midst of a perfect relationship with each other and their world, they lived in a pure love relationship with the Creator. A constant flow of communication, affection, and understanding streamed between God and His creatures through the indwelling of the human spirit. So great was their unity that Adam was said to be made in the very "image of God" Himself (Genesis 1: 26-27).

This was the original design. This was what God designed to be "normal." This was the intention of the Creator: *Man and woman, in full unity with God.* It was good. In fact it was "very good" (Genesis 1:31).

But it didn't last.

The "Fall" of Humanity

There was only one negative command in Eden; and daily the tempta-tion hung low from a nearby branch:

From any tree of the garden you may eat freely;
but from the tree of the knowledge of good and
evil you shall not eat, for in the day that
you eat from it you will surely die.
GENESIS 2:16-17

It doesn't seem like much of a lure in itself, particularly for those who had all abundance in eternal measure. But mixed with a lie from the lips of the Destroyer, the fragrance of the fruit began to waft in their souls:

You surely will not die!
For God knows that in the day you eat from it,
your eyes will be opened, and you will be like God,
knowing good and evil.
GENESIS 3:4-5

"You will be like God. You will be like God. You will be like God." Who knows for certain how the lie appealed to their mind or emotions? What lust did it ignite in their souls? All we know for sure is that the deception enticed them and carried them away, giving birth to sin, and when the sin was com-plete, it ushered in death (James 1:14-15).

They took a step away from the design, seeking to become more like God Himself, even though they were already like Him in many ways, having been made in God's image (Genesis 1:26). This decision has had devastat-ing earthly and eternal consequences for them and all of their descendents: Death.

First and foremost came spiritual death. The very life of God—His Spirit —left them. Now, instead of unity with God, humanity would forever be born spiritually dead, separate from the Creator—the only One who possesses the wisdom necessary to live life as designed. Like a tidal wave that devastates every shore of our being, this core spiritual problem has been the norm ever since. *We are born spiritually separated from the One who knows us and loves us most.*

Second, our souls now operate in a vacuum of truth and guidance. We can only navigate naturally, rather than supernaturally.

But a natural man does not accept the things
of the Spirit of God, for they are foolishness to him;
and he cannot understand them,
because they are spiritually appraised.
CORINTHIANS 2:14

We now choose good and evil based on what appeals to our souls and the urges of our bodies (which are continually stimulated and deceived by the world around us). Humanity has devised and created a vast array of devises to try to fill that vacuum—everything from religion to war—and yet the emptiness haunts us. On a grander scale, our societies are filled with masses who are doing what seems right in their own eyes... but the efforts lead only to more death (Proverbs 16:25). A more stress-filled environment could not exist.

Mental stress—a symptom of our attempts to be our own gods—is also destroying our bodies and our minds. The pressures of the modern world and our internal fight to find stability and purpose force our minds into chronic levels of anxiety in the best case scenarios and in the worst case scenarios, cause us to break down.

In the midst of it all we find ourselves in desperation. Trying whatever we can in our own strength, we search to find (even in the smallest measure) the purpose and peace that were so abundant in God's original plan. Our attempts, however, only make things worse; we become disheartened and disillusioned. Many face discouragement and depression daily.

Even the foods we eat have been severely compromised, lacking vital nutrients to sustain our bodies and provide the nutrients we need. Many of the foods available today are highly processed and low in nutritional value. Many foods are actually highly addictive, making us slaves and dragging us into the bondage of obesity and diabetes.

And finally, at the end of it all, each of us face the certainty of physical death (Genesis 3:17-19). Death may come in the instant of an "untimely" accident, through the pain and decay of disease, or at the "natural" end of a long life. But let there be no doubt: our heart will beat its last, our lungs will expel a final puff of air, and the blood will begin to cool in our veins... and our spirit and souls will enter eternity... either with or without the Spirit of God.

Spirit, Soul, and Body Are One

Clear distinctions can and should be made between spirit, soul, and body. At the same time however, these essential aspects of our humanity are intimately and inseparably connected.

> *For the word of God is living and active*
> *and sharper than any two-edged sword,*
> *and piercing as far as the division of soul and spirit,*
> *of both joints and marrow, and able to judge*
> *the thoughts and intentions of the heart.*
> HEBREWS 4:12

Bill and I have spent years counseling and treating individuals who have lost their health, their mind, or their peace. We have learned that a physical problem may present itself as a spiritual problem and vise versa (a spiritual problem can present as a physical problem). The mind, will, and emotion of the soul, while distinct, have inseparable impact on the spirit and the body. In order to help any client or patient it is critical that we correctly identify where the problem originates.

Jane's Story

Jane was tall and naturally attractive, but the first time she came into Bill's office, that attractiveness dissolved into a storm of distorted and fearful words. As her thoughts poured out, the root of her concerns was revealed: Jane was convinced that she was under spiritual attack. Her mind was being consumed with confusion, anger, and bitterness at a level she had never experienced before. Jane was not under any financial or outside emotional stress. She was a godly woman with a history of deep intimacy in her relationship with Christ. Over the past few months, however, that closeness with God seemed to evaporate, leaving her alone and desperate.

Bill saw her a couple of times, and together they walked through spiritual warfare issues and sorted through an assortment of beliefs and thoughts. Finding little to be concerned with, however, Bill began to wonder if the battle in Jane's soul might not have physical causes. Could there be something amiss in her body? He sent her to my office to find out.

When I first saw her, it was obvious to me that Jane was beginning to show signs of acute anxiety and depression. Tears began to flow as she described her attempts to control her thoughts, but she felt her mind was out of control. On top of that, she seemed to be living in condemnation and failure with her spiritual walk. As I performed a complete history and physical, I discovered that she was 46 years old and that her menstrual periods had started to become a little irregular. She really wasn't having any night sweats or hot flashes, but she was definitely noting mental confusion and uncontrollable mood swings, yet her lab work and her physical examination showed nothing abnormal. The diagnosis was not difficult to make: Jane was entering early menopause—what is referred to as the "perimenopausal time." I decided to give her a trial of low-dose, natural hormonal replacement to treat this physical condition rather than simply placing her on an antidepressant to treat the emotional and mental concerns.

I saw Jane in my office approximately four weeks later. During this visit, she described to me her near miraculous recovery. Within days of beginning the natural hormonal replacement she began feeling more like herself. Her anxiety began to settle down and her mind began to quit racing. Peace became a part of her life again and she felt God's involvement and care. In short, she had gotten her life back and she now feels perfectly normal. In my 30 plus years of practice, I have been involved with problems like Jane's many times. I have found that many women have more difficulty during their perimenopausal time (the three to four years before they actually go through menopause) than when they actually go through menopause. (Ovaries don't just quit making hormones all at once. They actually sputter as they slow down, causing hormones to vacillate more severely.) In Jane's case, *she didn't have a spiritual problem, but a physical problem that presented itself as a problem within her soul.*

Mark's Story

Mark had been a patient for years and had been in excellent health. A man of ambition and enthusiasm, his journey through life took an unexpected turn when he began suffering increasing amounts of pain in his joints, primarily in his knees, hands, and wrists—the red, swollen joints painfully tender to the touch. His blood work was negative for gout and negative for all forms of arthritis. Oddly, however, his test revealed a significant amount of inflammation in his body. Something was causing an acute flare-up of his joints, and I concluded that it was due to underlying osteoarthritis. I prescribed a basic nonsteroidal anti-inflammatory and followed him closely over the next couple of months. But nothing seemed to make a dent in his symptoms. I tried several different medications yet in some ways he actually was getting worse.

During one of our appointments, I decided to just sit and ask questions. As I did, the lid came off of Mark's life...and the contents weren't pretty. Inside Mark's soul swirled a cesspool of disappointment and frustration. First the failure of his marriage—the heartbreak of so many hopes and dreams. The divorce had resulted in an ongoing, gut-wrenching, child-custody dispute. There was far more going on than I could touch medically, and I suggested Mark spend some time with Bill.

Over the next weeks, Mark and Bill walked together along a difficult path. Time and time again, they confronted Mark's anger...anger that had been allowed to simmer and brew, eventually consuming, controlling, and dominating his life. From the Scriptures, Bill led Mark through the principles of true biblical forgiveness. Hurting enough to take the counseling seriously, Mark spent many hours in God's Word and in prayer, completing the assignments that Bill had given him. Issue by issue Mark was set free from the bitter heart that had been imprisoning him.

Then, to Mark's amazement (and mine), he began noting significant improvement in his physical health. His joints—so wracked with pain before—became progressively less and less tender. Within five or six weeks his joints returned to normal. Mark had totally stopped any medication when he began seeing Bill, so we knew that something else had prompted his healing. The only conclusion was obvious: Mark had had a problem in his soul, and the stress it was causing was destroying his body. Mark continues to walk a path of forgiveness and has been totally free of any joint pain or inflammation for over two years now.

Your Story

Like Jane and Mark, you too are made up of a spirit, soul, and body; many parts, but all members of one body, all interconnected and affecting each other. Paul understood the integration of the human body, and used it as an analogy of the way the church ought to function.

For just as we have many members in one body
and all the members do not have the same function,
so we, who are many, are one body in Christ,
and individually members one of another.
ROMANS 12:4-5

But God has so composed the body, giving more
abundant honor to that member which lacked,
so that there may be no division in the body, but that the
members should have the same care for one another.
And if one member suffers, all the members suffer with it;
if one member is honored, all the members rejoice with it.
1 CORINTHIANS 12:24-27

When you are having problems with one of the parts of your being, it will definitely affect the others. If you have a spiritual problem, it can affect both your soul and body. Likewise, a physical problem can also affect your soul. Identifying where the problem is primarily rooted is an essential aspect for restoring your health and peace. Understanding this interconnectedness is clearly essential to fulfilling your call to present yourself complete to God.

Yes, in the beginning, God created the heavens and the earth...and He created you as well. Your body, soul, and spirit are of His design...a design that reflects the creative power of God Himself, a design that illuminates His original intent for how we are to live both now and in eternity.

As we look through the lenses of both Scripture and science, Bill and I pray that your eyes will be opened to see not only the challenges that the spirit, soul, and body face in this fallen world but also that freedom and worship might be ignited as His truth comes alive in *all three* aspects of your being. We will begin with the universal experience of "stress," then move on to other aspects of life that impact us. Our desire is that, in the end, you might love Him more—with all your spirit, soul, and body—as long as He gives you breath upon this earth...and then for an eternity to follow.

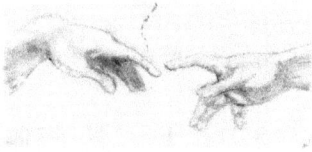

CHAPTER 2

Stress

"Therefore do not be anxious for tomorrow;

for tomorrow will care for itself.

Each day has enough trouble of its own."

MATTHEW 6:34

Part 1: ALL STRESSED OUT

Michael is a vice president of a struggling company. He has worked for this position since college, but the large desk in the corner office is not what he dreamed it would be. Stuck between the CEO and the managers, his life is a conduit of complaints and concerns from the top to the bottom, and the bottom to the top. A martini at lunch helps him get through the afternoon, but long after he gets home in the evening, spread sheets and cash flow analysis continue to ravish his mind.

David is a pastor. It's late Saturday night and he is still at the keyboard, trying to complete the outline for his sermon. In his thoughts he sees the faces in the congregation, his board of elders, and his seminary professors. He feels them looking over his shoulder at his work; he imagines them in the pews the next morning, critiquing each word he says ... or worse yet, he sees them gazing at him with annoyed indifference. A familiar knot grows in his stomach. He tries to focus on the Bible; he tries to pray, but his concentration is stolen away by the faces he sees.

Linda is a soccer mom. From dawn to dusk, her day is maze of carpools, cleaning, and grocery stores. She drives with a cell phone cocked to her ear, trying to maintain contact with key customers for her home-based business. At the moment, she is on her way to a church planning meeting, where women with perfect makeup will expound on all the extra activities that they do for their children, bringing such growth to their mental, emotional, and spiritual lives. Tonight when the kids are at last in bed and the last of the dishes are dry, her exhausted body will collapse in bed with her husband. Will there be anything left to give him when he turns out the lights? She doubts it, and anticipates the coolness of his disappointment.

Michael, David, and Linda: What do they all have in common? *Stress.* Emotional and mental stress pushes them into anxiety and worry. These emotions (unbeknownst to them) are also causing destructive damage in their bodies. What else do they have in common? *They are probably a lot like you.* Sure, the circumstances might be different, but the stress they feel is not unlike yours.

The dictionary defines stress as "a mentally or emotionally disruptive or disquieting influence; or distress." Stress is any type of situation that places conflicting or heavy demands upon a person's mind, emotions, or body. These demands upset the body's normal equilibrium and create "stress." Our bodies respond to stress by releasing excessive amounts of "stress hormones" such as adrenaline, noradrenaline, and cortisol. The greater the physical or emotional stress, the greater the stimulation and release of these stress hormones.

Cortisol levels, for example, increase dramatically within minutes, whether the stress is physical (trauma, shock, severe exercise, surgery), psychological (anxiety, panic, depression), or physiologic (low blood sugar, fever). Elevated cortisol levels are necessary to protect the body when it is under stress. As part of God's design, cortisol was created to protect us in our greatest time of need, during those minutes when our lives are at serious risk.

Cortisol raises blood sugar, suppresses insulin levels, and decreases inflammation by directly inhibiting or depressing the immune system. Rising levels of adrenaline increase blood pressure, pulse rate, and respiratory rate. That's okay for a few minutes or maybe even an hour, but when stress becomes a chronic or recurring issue, major medical problems can arise. My personal experience is that severe and chronic stress is the main reason many of my patients are becoming ill and requiring medical attention. Symptoms of stress are a primary reason people come to Bill's counseling center. Neither the body nor the soul was designed to handle severe or prolonged stress. The stress response was designed for something entirely different.

> **My personal experience is that severe and chronic stress is the main reason many of my patients are becoming ill and requiring medical attention.**

Fight or Flight Response

When our conscious mind senses an eminent danger, whether real or imagined, God designed us to respond quickly and abruptly. There is a tremendous release of our stress hormones that almost immediately begin to do their work. Our pulse rate jumps and we may even feel our heart beating strongly in our chest. Our breathing increases and we may get sweaty palms and even shaking hands. Our muscle tone increases as we are ready to respond quickly for any action. This intense response is referred to as the "fight or flight" response. After our conscious mind evaluates the threat, our will then chooses either to fight or flee the situation.

Normally, the stressful episode passes fairly rapidly and our bodies and thoughts return to a more normal state. This is the way we were designed to experience the stress reaction. It was created to protect us in our time of greatest need. However, in today's world, we are repeatedly stimulating this protective stress reaction because of the way we are choosing to live our lives.

Sources of Stress in Our Lives

Have you ever really stopped to think about the amount of stress you face in your day-to-day lives? You have probably grown to accept it as the "norm"—as an undesirable but unavoidable aspect of existence. But excessive, chronic stress is not normal—and I think you would be shocked by how it impacts your peace and your joy... as well as your health.

Our lives are filled with all kinds of commitments, obligations, duties, and noise. We have worry about our spouse, our children, our finances, our job, our health, and our future. No wonder we cannot hear the soft voice of God whispering to our soul! No wonder peace seems so illusive. Stress and anxiety are part of living—*but the way we handle it is robbing us of peace, joy, and health.* Stress is the opposite of peace. As Christians we are offered a peace that surpasses all comprehension (Philippians 4:7). Yet it seems that Christians struggle with stress as much as (or even more than) others. Why is that? What are the circumstances that continually push us over the edge?

Financial Pressure

In today's world, I feel that one of the greatest causes of stress and pressure comes from financial worries and concerns. We are bombarded by marketing gurus every time we turn on our TVs, look in the newspaper, or read a magazine. The merchants of materialism spend billions of dollars a year stimulating our desires and felt needs for more and more. Left unchecked by God's truth, our "desires" quickly become "needs." (In our minds we become convinced that we *must* have them in order to have joy and fulfillment.) We need that beautiful home in the perfect location along with a two or three car garage and beautiful cars to fill them. We must have the newest technology when it comes to our televisions, computers, video cameras, and stereos. We need the latest fashions, most beautiful jewelry and cosmetics.

Not only do we feel we need everything that is available around us, but also we feel we need it *now*. Forget about saving diligently for something special that you want; your mailbox is full of messages from corporations who are willing to give you all the credit you need to get what you want today. Why wait? We can have what we want immediately, deferring payment indefinitely. But as easy short-term credit adds up, even the smallest change in your monthly income—or one unexpected expense—can place you in an immediate crisis.

The truth of the matter is that our lifestyles often control our lives. How much time do you think about or worry about financial problems? Do your financial obligations drive you to work longer hours or get that second job? More importantly, does the financial stress and pressure you have placed on yourself affect your relationships with your spouse, family, loved ones, and friends? Have finances become a barrier for having a more, intimate relationship with your Creator? Are you anxious about tomorrow, wondering whether you will have enough money this month to pay your bills?

Time Pressures, Over Commitment, and Deadlines

Most of us are our own worst enemies when it comes to creating insanely hurried lives. The choices we make and the dreams we chase fill our schedules to the brim. Often our commitments drain us of every available moment and every ounce of spare energy. The days are packed and so are the weekends. Saturdays are packed with chores and sports. Getting to church on Sunday can be one of the most stressful events in a family's week. (So much for the "day of rest!") Transporting children to piano lessons, gymnastics, baseball, soccer, basketball practice, or the school play can be a full-time job all by itself. Competition and the need to have our children succeed in any and every aspect of their lives drive parents beyond any logic. Hurried lives keep us on the run, never affording us the chance to live in the here-and-now, and never giving opportunity to rest and listen to God.

Perfectionism

Do you live with the feeling that you're never doing quite *enough* or not doing it *well* enough? The very foundation of Western society is based on the belief that *a person's value comes from what they have, what they do, and what they look like.* Each time we act on that belief, we are catapulted into a stressful cycle that quickly begins to spiral out of control. When we become absorbed with our performance, appearance, and possessions everything has to be "just right." When it's not, our personal value gets thrown into question, exposing us to rejection. The only way to succeed at the performance-perfectionism game is to give 100 percent, and to give it 100 percent of the time. Still we fear that our best isn't good enough, and the fear saps us of our energy, our time...and sometimes our integrity. Unfortunately, organized religion does little to help relieve this pressure. More often than not, it adds to the pressure by adding more activity, more pressure, and more judgment.

The demand to perform can also turn us into control freaks. Perfectionism often causes us to try to manipulate circumstances and the people around us (particularly those closest to us, such as our spouse or kids). That causes even *more* stress, because people and circumstance are not ours to control. That was never part of the design—yet we try to do it all the time.

Operating Outside of Our Gifts and Talents

God has created each of us in unique ways for unique purposes, and He's given each of us specific gifts and skills to fulfill these purposes. When we work within these gifts and talents, our efforts seem to come naturally and easily.

For we are His workmanship,
created in Christ Jesus for good works,
which God prepared beforehand,
so that we would walk in them.
EPHESIANS 2:10

From time to time, we need to be stretched out of our "comfort zones" and pushed into new challenges. That stretching is healthy and therapeutic as it expands our horizons and helps us to discover new things about ourselves and about God. Many of us, however, find ourselves involved with tasks we aren't good at and often detest. It happens at work when we are promoted beyond our area of competency or when the boss is always asking for a little more. It happens at church when we fall prey to the "must-fill-the-need" mentality and get pressured into doing things that are outside our gifting and skills. If we don't respond to the need, we usually feel guilty, and that only adds more mental stress.

Projecting into the Future

God designed us to be concerned about the here-and-now, promising only enough faith to get us through this day:

So do not worry about tomorrow;
for tomorrow will care for itself.
Each day has enough trouble of its own.
MATTHEW 6:34

Yet don't we all become concerned, worried, and overwhelmed by what tomorrow might bring or not bring? At Bill's counseling center, they call it "The 'What If ____' Syndrome." Fill in the blank with anything you want: war, broken relationships, an overdrawn bank account, illness, death, a car crash, a deviant child, rain, no rain, etc. Let's face it; anything could happen tomorrow. If we try to live there and worry about things that probably won't happen anyway, the concerns attack our bodies and souls with undo stress.

Projecting into the unknown future, coupled with an uncertain conviction about the character of God, propels many of us into chronic levels of stress. A significant amount of emotional and mental stress emerges from concerns about the future.

Relationships

Perhaps our greatest source of emotional stress is interpersonal relationships. Relationships are like an intricate and delicate dance, requiring constant attention as they change to the beat of different music. Sometimes there is harmony, but often there is tension. When relationships lose their rhythm, toes get stepped on. And isn't it interesting that those we love the most have the greatest power to hurt us and the ones we desire to please the most often seem to be the most critical? Broken expectations, desires that go unfulfilled, accidental misunderstandings, and intentional wounds all cause us stress. If we think that we are responsible for other people's happiness or contentment, our stress levels can jump significantly.

If we think that we are responsible for other people's happiness or contentment, our stress levels can jump significantly.

Left to our own instincts and the examples of others, we deal with relationships as best we can. In the end, people let us down, we let them down, and conflict never gets resolved quite like it does on a 30-minute sitcom. And that causes lots of stress because many of us believe that it's our responsibility to make others happy. Many of us instinctively feel that our happiness is dependent on others being happy with us. Bill calls that "relational idolatry," and it results from us focusing on ourselves and others as our primary source of meaning, acceptance, and joy. Again, that's contrary to the design. God alone is to be the focus of that kind of attention (and thankfully, He is fully worthy of it!).

Many of us have spent our entire lives trying to please others. Never being able to say "no" may be one of your most serious problems. You obligate yourself and your precious spare time to make someone else happy with you but once you have made the commitment, you realize the additional stress this is going to place on yourself and your family. "Relational idolatry" may look good on the surface. From the outside it might make you look like a sacrificial father, a dedicated wife, or an active servant of God. But inside, concern about self and others is very stressful and can become a barrier to our most important commitment: developing a close, intimate relationship with our Lord and Savior.

Noise

"Noise" comes in many forms. Urban life is saturated with "noise pollution" and our homes and offices are filled with the sounds of people, radios, machinery, toys, and TVs. Beyond physical noise lies the concerns of *mental* noise and *emotional* noise, as each affect the body and the soul as directly as physical noise. Mental noise originates in our minds and then seeps into every aspect of our being. Thoughts about our schedules, our plans, our dreams and desires; thoughts about our health, our finances and our careers swirl in our heads and hearts all day long, eating up huge amounts of physical and mental energy.

Emotional noise (particularly from anger) consumes our energies and stimulates the stress response as well. Feelings of dejectedness, extended sorrow, and frustration spark numerous chemical stress reactions in the body, causing heightened levels of stress hormones. Physical pain is also a powerful stressor, directly stressing the body and indirectly fueling the stress response through mental concerns.

Perhaps the most serious aspect of stress from noise, however, is that it can drown out the persistent (but quiet) voice of the Holy Spirit and God's Word. When these channels of communication with the Creator are strained, we become isolated from everything that is absolutely essential for long-term victory over stress.

(For a more thorough discussion of this topic, see Chapter 3 of *Rest Assured,* by Bill Ewing, Real Life Press, 2003.)

Fear

Fear of danger, fear of pain, fear of loss, fear of rejection, fear of injury, fear of failure.... the fear of *anything* can trigger the stress reaction. Even the *expectation* of danger, pain, illness, or loss can send shock waves of stress through our bodies. When our minds perceive something is to be feared, our bodies launch the fight-or-flight stress response.

Many of our fears are learned and inherited from our families, friends, schools, and education. Our parents' fears are likely to become our own, and our fears are likely to be passed on to our children. We learn from the evening news and weekend movies to fear many things: spiders, terrorism, snakes, fire, heights, robbery, or abuse. The potential list is endless. *Anything* can cause fear if we think that it might be a real threat to the things we hold dear.

Fear can come from a past traumatic experience that has been permanently seared into the memory banks of the brain. Simply remembering a particular experience can repeatedly set off the same stress reaction that you originally had when the event occurred—even though there is no current threat of the same danger. Sometimes a similar circumstance triggers the stress response, as the mind makes a connection between something that happened in the past and something that could happen again, right now.

Uncontrolled fears can also become phobias. This consuming concern for germs, confined space, water, or solitude can lead to obsessive-compulsive behaviors that take control of our lives. It is critical to realize that not only our fears but also our thoughts, our concerns, our worries, and even our memories are capable of setting off this stress response, which can destroy our peace and joy, and also our physical health.

Anxiety and Panic Attacks

If unchecked by truth, fear can escalate into full-blown anxiety attacks and uncontrollable panic, bringing life to a chaotic, paralyzing stop. The same circumstances can also lead to depression. Why are some people prone to anxiety and some to depression? It's not always easy to tell, but often it has to do with issues of control. A person who is more passive will tend to get depressed and debilitated. A person with a controlling demeanor often thrives on stress, but when they feel they are loosing control they move into anxiety and then panic.

Many anxieties come from thoughts about events that are not happening (and probably never will happen). But the body doesn't know the difference and reacts as if the event were actually taking place. Stress hormones are released, causing high levels of tension and feelings of being out of control. Panic attacks are both the *result* of an excessive release of stress hormones and the *cause* of excessive stress hormones. It is a vicious cycle, and once you are in a panic attack it is very difficult to gain control of your thoughts. Pulse rates jump for no reason. Hands break out into a sweat. Often, it's difficult to breath and the mouth gets dry. You can even experience chest pain or the feeling that you are dying.

These symptoms make it difficult for a person to capture their thoughts, making them feel as if they've totally lost control—and that there is no escaping this horrifying state. Panic and anxiety attacks can incapacitate us mainly because we can't control this reaction. Lawyers, ministers, high performing business people, mothers... all are susceptible.

The unique thing about a panic attack is the fact that the patient some-times has no idea what is setting it off. Oftentimes they don't have any conscious thoughts of anxiety or fear. But once a panic attack begins, they have no way of stopping it and they can even feel as if they are going to die. The experience is truly indescribable. You can't relate to it unless you've been there. Some describe it as running on 220 volts when you are wired for 110. One patient described it this way:

> I feel like I'm in another world.
> It's like I know I'm there, but I'm really not.
> I feel removed from the situation I'm in.
> I feel like I'm in another dimension—like a
> hollow or vacuum—outside the situation.
> It's like watching the whole thing from a distance.

A World War II veteran, who had participated in one of the first troop waves to land on the Normandy beaches on D-Day said this about his anxiety attacks:

> The fear I felt landing on the beaches
> was mild compared to the sheer terror of a bad panic attack.
> Given the choice between the two, I would gladly
> again volunteer to land in Normandy.

Yes, stress is an unavoidable component of life, and God designed us to be able to handle it in short-term "fight or flight" situations. But the body and soul were never designed for the chronic, ongoing stress that begins in our mind and then sends shock waves through our being. Scripture calls us to be aware of the thoughts that cause this kind of stress. Consider the following from Psalm 139:23-24:

> Search me, O God, and know my heart;
> try me and know my anxious thoughts;
> and see if there be any hurtful way in me,
> and lead me in the everlasting way.

In the pages ahead, we will look more in-depth at the ravaging effects of stress on the body. But for now, I would strongly encourage you to take sometime and make the prayer of Psalm 139 your own. Ask God to search your heart, to show you your anxious thoughts, to reveal the hurt that these thoughts are causing you and those around you...and then ask Him to lead you into a life that deals with stress according to His design, rather than contrary to it. Ask and He will begin to lead you into a "way" of living that will last forever. Ask, and through His Word and His Spirit, I believe He will answer.

Part 2: THE MIND/BODY CONNECTION

Over the past half century, a tremendous amount of research has shown how important our mind and our thoughts are to our overall physical health. Much of what happens in the body begins in our mind. Our thoughts and emotions have a tremendous influence on our body. We have been discussing the stress reaction that occurs as a normal, protective response to danger or serious injury to our body. This reaction was designed by God for our safety and protection and is a critical aspect of health.

Hopefully you are beginning to appreciate the fact that this same response can also be elicited by our thoughts, concerns, memories, fears, and worries. When you become anxious about anything, your anxious thoughts actually stimulate this stress reaction within your body. Therefore, what is happening in your mind has a tremendous influence on your physical body.

Each time our conscious mind senses danger, the unconscious mind triggers this fight or flight stress response. Each time your pulse rate and respiratory rate increases, blood pressure rises, blood sugar rises, and the immune system is suppressed. Each time there is an excessive release of these stress hormones. If these anxious thoughts are handled according to God's Word, this reaction will settle down fairly quickly and there is really no negative effect on our bodies. However, if we do not deal with the thoughts appropriately, it can lead to a prolonged or chronic stress reaction that can potentially cause serious damage to our health. If stress is prolonged, the protective stress response—a vital short-term defense mechanism—actually now becomes our enemy.

Oxidative Stress—the "Dark Side" of Oxygen

One of the damaging aspects of prolonged or repeated bouts of stress is a different kind of stress, called "oxidative stress." This type of stress attacks the body from *within,* robbing us of our health.

Oxygen is essential for life itself, however, it is also inherently dangerous for our existence. As you utilize oxygen within the furnace of the cell (called the "mitochondria"), occasionally a "free radical" or charged oxygen molecule is produced. A free radical is an oxygen molecule that has at least one unpaired electron in its outer orbit. This gives an oxygen molecule an electrical charge and causes it to move very rapidly. If this charged oxygen molecule is not readily neutralized by an "antioxidant," it can go on to damage the cell wall, vessel wall, proteins, fats, and even the DNA of the cell.

Oxidative stress has been shown in medical literature to be the root cause of over 70 chronic degenerative diseases. These are diseases such as heart attacks, strokes, cancer, diabetes, Alzheimer's dementia, Parkinson's disease, arthritis, macular degeneration, multiple sclerosis, lupus...and the list goes on and on. (I have written about oxidative stress and its risk to our bodies and health in my book, *What Your Doctor Doesn't Know about Nutritional Medicine* (Thomas Nelson 2002). I would encourage you to pick up a copy and read it if you would like to know more about this subject.

A good illustration that explains how oxidative stress damages our bodies is a wood fireplace. Ninety-five percent of the time the wood fire burns just fine. However, occasionally there is a "pop," and out jumps a hot cinder that burns a little hole in your carpet. That is really not too big of a problem; but if it continues month after month and year after year, you'll end up with pitted, frayed, and ratty carpet. Look at the fireplace as the furnace of your cell (mitochondria) and the cinder as the occasional free radical it produces. The carpet is your body.

The disease you may develop will be determined by the part of the body that wears out first. If it is the brain, you could develop Parkinson's disease or Alzheimer's dementia. If it is your arteries, you could suffer a heart attack or stroke. If it is your joints, you could develop arthritis. If it is your eyes, you could develop a cataract or macular degeneration. The process (oxidation) that causes a cut apple to turn brown or metal to rust is the same process that can cause all of the diseases listed above. Diseases you and I would love to avoid. Oxidative stress can cause you to simply rust inside.

We are not defenseless against the onslaught of free radicals, however. "Antioxidants" have the ability to give up an electron to a free radical and render it harmless, acting like the glass doors or fine wire mesh that we put in front of our fireplaces. The sparks will still fly, however, the carpet (your body) is protected. God designed the body to make some of the antioxidants we need. We also get some antioxidants from our foods—especially from fruits and vegetables. Vitamin C, vitamin E, beta carotene, alpha lipoic acid, and glutathione are some examples of antioxidants.

It's All about Balance

Controlling oxidative stress is all about balance. If you have enough antioxidants available to neutralize all the free radicals you produce, there will be no damage. However, if you are producing more free radicals than your body can neutralize, you will suffer oxidative stress. If this occurs for a prolonged period of time, it can cost you your health and even your life. Consuming high-quality, complete, and balanced nutritional supplements provides the body with the micronutrients it needs to optimize the body's natural antioxidant defense system, natural immune system, and natural repair system. Providing the body with nutritional supplements, allows the body to function the way God designed it. (Nutritional supplements are discussed in more detail in Chapter 9.)

The number of free radicals you and I produce in any given day is not constant. A certain amount of free radical production occurs by just metabolizing our food to create energy. However, the pollutants in our air, food, and water significantly increase the number of free radicals the body produces. When you exercise mildly or moderately, the number of free radicals you produce goes up just a little. However, if you *over* exercise, free radical levels go up exponentially, right off the chart. Cigarette smoke, radiation, sunlight, and medication also increase the number of free radicals.

Surprisingly, the greatest cause of increased free radical production is emotional stress. If you have short-term stress (or even mild to moderate stress) the number of free radicals you produce goes up only a little. The body can normally handle this mild increase very easily. However, if you are under severe or prolonged stress, the number of free radicals you produce goes up exponentially. This is the main reason that recurrent or prolonged stress and anxiety can cause such devastation to our bodies—*if it is not handled according to God's design.* I personally believe that stress which is not dealt with according to God's direction is one of the main reasons that we are dealing with so much chronic degenerative disease in our world today.

Time magazine ran an article called "The Ravages of Stress" (December 13, 2004) summarizing a report in *The Proceedings of the National Academy of Sciences.* A team of scientists reported that long-term, unrelenting stress on mothers (who were caring for seriously disabled children) led to premature aging of their cells. These mothers cared for children with cerebral palsy, autism, and other serious disorders. Compared to mothers of less demanding children, they had much higher levels of free radical produc-

Now researchers have been able to show what we all have known instinctively for years: *Chronic stress weakens the immune system, raises the risk of chronic degenerative disease, and even causes premature death.*

tion and oxidative stress. The researchers were able to show that oxidative stress caused significant damage to their cells and their genes.

As a physician, I'm always concerned for individuals who are suffering from major chronic degenerative disease, but I'm often *more* concerned for the spouse who is the caregiver. I can't tell you the number of times I witnessed a caregiver who died before their debilitated spouse. Now researchers have been able to show what we all have known instinctively for years: *Chronic stress weakens the immune system, raises the risk of chronic degenerative disease, and even causes premature death.*

I am sure that you can remember a time in your life that you experienced unusual or prolonged stress and came down with a severe cold, pneumonia, or other acute illness. You may even recall a loved one who was under severe and prolonged stress who suffered their first heart attack, stroke, or even cancer. High levels of stress hormones along with excessive free radicals are the reasons this occurs.

Oxidative Stress Leads to Inflammation

Unfortunately, the bad news doesn't end there. Another result of elevated stress hormones and free radicals in our body is "destructive inflammation." Once free radicals injure the body, our natural immune system is called in to try and repair that damage. Normally, the immune system is our great protector. It continuously seeks out and identifies foreign objects, viruses, bacteria, or abnormally growing cells which it normally destroys quickly. *Interestingly, the immune system actually produces free radicals,* which it then uses to destroy these invaders. If the battle is won, the level of free radicals returns to normal. (That's the good side of oxidative stress and the immune system: It is a key weapon needed to protect our health.) However, there is a bad side to oxidative stress and the immune system. It's very much like "friendly fire" in a war—when the weapons of our allies are accidentally turned against us, causing injury and death.

The immune system creates an inflammatory response to repair an injury. ("Inflammation" is redness and swelling at the point of damage.) If the immune system does not shut itself off, the excessive free radicals it produces can actually lead to *more* damage. As the inflammatory response caused by the immune system attempts to repair the damage created by oxidative stress, it causes even more free radicals in the process. As this cycle continues, a "low-grade, chronic inflammatory response" occurs—especially if there is ongoing oxidative stress. Therefore, recurring or chronic stress can not only suppress and attack our immune system, but also it can eventually lead to the serious chronic degenerative diseases all of us would like to avoid.

Remember, it is all about balance! You want to have enough antioxidants on board to handle the number of free radicals you produce. If you don't, free radicals will win battle after battle. When the war is over, you don't get to choose your conqueror. All you will know is that a serious "chronic degenerative disease" has set up an occupation in your body and now seeks total domination.

The Result: Burnout, Breakdown, or Decay

Stress hormones are stored in the adrenal glands and at the nerve endings and are quickly released into the body during times of stress. An individual who is under chronic stress or repeated severe stress may develop significant and serious depletion of their stress hormones. Usually my patients are not even aware that this is happening until it is too late. They come into my office completely exhausted, severely fatigued, and experiencing what most of us refer to as "burnout."

The human body is worn down by stress just as a battery operated radio or TV is worn down by continued use. The radio operates normally—even though the batteries are being run down over time. You don't even think about it until all of sudden one day there are a few moments of static and then "poof," the radio or TV just doesn't work. The human body responds in a similar way. We continue to live our stressful lives normally until we finally just tip over into total exhaustion and burnout. This often happens without warning, or at least very little of it.

God's Peace

The God-given body-soul-spirit design is being attacked on all fronts by stress. So vital is this issue that a significant portion of the Bible addresses the connection between stress, anxiety, and physical health:

> *For this reason I say to you, do not be anxious for your life,*
> *as to what you shall eat, or what you shall drink;*

nor for your body, as to what you shall put on ...
And which of you by being anxious can add a single
cubit to his life's span? And why are you anxious about clothing?
... Do not be anxious then, saying, "What shall we eat?"
or "What shall we drink?" or "With what shall we clothe ourselves?"
... But seek first His kingdom and His righteousness;
and all these things shall be added to you. Therefore do not
be anxious for tomorrow; for tomorrow will care for itself.
Each day has enough trouble of its own.

MATTHEW 6:25, 27-28, 33-34

Be anxious for nothing, but in everything by prayer
and supplication with thanksgiving let your requests
be made known to God. And the peace of God,
which surpasses all comprehension,
will guard your hearts and your minds in Christ Jesus.

PHILIPPIANS 4:6-7

What Can Be Done?

Changing your circumstances can help *reduce* stress, and in many situations (within biblical parameters), I highly recommend that you do so. But be honest; you've probably tried this in the past and found temporary relief at best. Stressful circumstances are a part of life in this fallen world, and you can't change very many of them. More importantly, stress is a *response* that is triggered by circumstances, but originates in the *mind.* You can change circumstances all you want, but the core problem of stress is in *you,* not "out there."

If you focus your heart on clear commands from God, and try to obey them with all your might, will it relieve stress? With all due respect to the infallible Word of God and your heartfelt effort, I have to tell you the truth: *It won't.* In fact, you will probably make things worse. Not only will you still be stressed, but also your inability to obey these commands of Scripture *on your own* will make you feel more guilty—and therefore, even more stressed out—because now you feel like a spiritual failure too.

This is my key point: We don't need to be reminded of *what* we are supposed to do or not do. *The problem is that we don't know how to do it.* We already know that stress is bad for us and a direct disobedience to the commands of the Bible. But small adjustments and more determination will not break the bondage of stress. A radical transformation must take place in the soul in order to relieve stress on the mind and the body.

A Complete Paradigm Shift

You can make significant changes in your circumstances, and you can earnestly try to obey Scripture with all your might. Do so and your life will be the better for it...maybe, for a little while. But the core issues of stress in all its forms are rooted much, much more strongly than that. The issues have to do with design. The issues have to do with belief. The issues have to do with central issues of the soul and the spirit.

> To find the peace, purpose, and health that God offers in lasting measure, we need to go deep. Band-Aids will not stick. Dealing with surface symptoms will not suffice.

To find the peace, purpose, and health that God offers in lasting measure, we need to go deep. Band-Aids will not stick. Dealing with surface symptoms will not suffice. A focus on the commands of Scripture without understanding the biblical context in which the command was given will always fail. We need more than a superficial understanding of what God desires and what we hope for. We need to diligently consider the biblical principles that reveal *how* we are to pursue His call upon our spirit, soul, and body. In the lines of the living Word of God we find the truths about *how* we were created, and how we are to live this life by His design—even in the midst of a fallen world, full of fleshly pain and failure.

Be forewarned: What He reveals is, in most cases, absolutely contrary to conventional wisdom. If you were hoping for simple inward adjustments that might make complex changes in your outward life, this is not the message for you. If you are willing to allow God Himself to make a complete paradigm shift in your inner soul—even if it appears to have little immediate effect on your outward circumstances—then "the peace of God, which surpasses all comprehension, will guard your hearts and your minds in Christ Jesus" (Philippians 4:7).

> *These things I have spoken to you,*
> *so that in Me you may have peace.*
> *In the world you have tribulation, but take courage,*
> *I have overcome the world.*
> JESUS CHRIST, JOHN 16:33

Reclaiming the Original Design

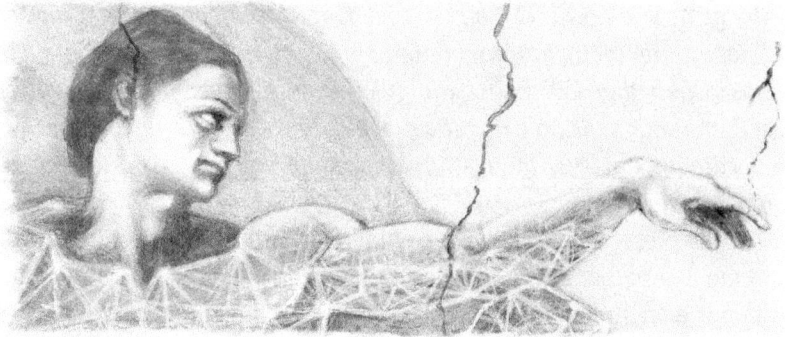

With hearts of stone and laws written upon the same, *God's most magnificent creations wandered for thousands of years, searching for hope, searching for stability, searching for anything to fill the nothingness that enveloped their spirits. Diligently they looked for anything to relieve the stressful pressure on their souls. Desperately they searched for answers that would shine a light beyond the grave...*

Then... again... from across the expanse of time and space, God spoke anew. Where He had first spoken by the resounding words of the universe's creation, this time He spoke through the womb of a simple woman. This time He didn't send a message, this time He became the message. The One "through whom all things came into being," became one of those beings Himself. "The Word became flesh, and dwelt among us, and we saw His glory ... full of grace and truth" (John 1:14). This time He came "... that they may have life, and have it abundantly" (John 10:10).

During the years His feet walked this earth, He spoke pointed truths about reconciliation, love, and a great hope in eternity. At His touch the sick found healing, the dead found new life, and the sinner found compassionate embrace.

Then, contrary to expectation—but in fulfillment of the prophecies of old—He intentionally walked a path that led Him to a hill outside of Jerusalem. There, with His flesh nailed to rough beams of wood, He willingly gave Himself as a perfect sacrifice for the sins of humans. Through His blood, those who were far off—those who were separated from the Creator by the things they had done and the things they had left undone—could find all things new: a new birth, a new covenant, a new hope for eternity.

Today, into the hollow void of the human spirit He now whispers an invitation: "Open the door and I will fill the nothingness again. I will speak Myself into your heart, making it a place of my habitation once more...where we, together, can savor the lost intimacy and love, and begin to reclaim the Grand Design."

In the preceding pages, I have written about the problems: the stress, the pain, the illness, and the frustration we feel when we try to live the Christian life in our own strength. Now we have reached a major turning point in this book. Perhaps it will be a turning point in your life as well. Bill and I want you to know that the things we will talk about in the next chapters revolutionized our faith, and we offer them to you with humility and sincerity. As a physician and a counselor, we will lay out to you, as best we can, some of the most powerful principles we know for reclaiming God's design.

To those of you who have been trying to live the Christian life—and found it wanting—we are baiting you with the hope that there is something different that you have missed, something that you can yet find that will free you from chronic concerns and stress. To those of you who find yourself on the edge of a new faith in Christ, we pray that these words will be used by Him to show you the way into a new relationship with your Creator, where you will come to know the forgiveness, the acceptance, and the indwelling presence of God Himself.

But we can take it only so far. In order for any of what follows to take root, we need the touch of the Master Physician and the words of the Mighty Counselor to reveal what is true and what is right. Our natural instincts, past experiences (and maybe even our current understanding of the Bible's core messages) can't take us there. God's Spirit and His Word must speak to us in new ways.

May God in His mercy and grace, touch our hearts to make His Word new and real today, and each day hereafter.

Master Designer,

We are at the end of our resources, and we need more. We have exhausted our understanding, and we still can't figure it out. We have tried as best we know how, and can't seem to make it work. Father, would You speak to us in a new way? Right now? Would You soften our tired and hardened hearts and show us a better way? We need Your Truth, and You must reveal it to us if we are to truly live by Your design.

Lord, we open our hearts to You now, perhaps for the first time, perhaps out of hunger for more of who You can be in our lives. Thank You for revealing Yourself through the creation and Your Word. Thank You for choosing the Cross and for sacrificing Yourself for our sins. We thank You for coming into our hearts and making us new.

Would You open our eyes now to the truths in Your Word that You have given to comfort, guide, and protect us? We need Your Spirit to speak that we might be able to hear and understand the way You have prepared for us to live. Give us clarity of thought. Protect us from the distractions and lies of evil.

Renew our minds and align them to the wonderful ways of Your perfect design.

Amen

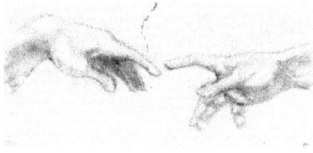

CHAPTER 3

Motivation of the Heart

The Christian life is rarely what it appears to be, and only infrequently is it what we desire it to be. Promises and commands of peace and harmony abound, but frustration often comes after we make that sincere commitment to follow Christ and commit our lives to Him—and then continue to face so much anxiety, stress, and unresolved anger in our lives. Even though we know that we have experienced the spiritual rebirth and have received His love and forgiveness, our lives are still filled with tremendous stress and anxiety. Where is that peace that we so much desire and want? You've probably tried hard to please God and to live the way He wants you to live, however, it just doesn't seem to be working. You want to be walking in His Spirit and experiencing His peace and fruits of the Spirit, however, you always seem to end up back where you started, flailing in your thoughts and actions. Where is the relief to this struggle? Where is the victory?

In the next four chapters we will answer those questions with sincerity and honesty. If you are looking for a formula that will be your quick fix to all your problems, you will walk away disappointed. If you are searching for a new paradigm (an entirely new way of thinking) that could entirely change *how* you live the Christian life, then you will find that God's holy and complete Word has much to say to your stress-ridden body and soul.

The Problem—the Trap of Self-Effort

We've established that a human being is made up of a spirit, soul, and body (with the soul being made up of your mind, will, and emotions). Prior to Christ coming into your life, those three parts interacted in a certain way, and they did so by "default" according to the way they were conditioned by influences of the world. Although your spirit has been made new, your body and soul may still function under these automatic, default settings. Your intellect and emotions control your will (which is the part of the soul that makes all decisions), and the will then determines your actions.

The world system measures our worth by our *performance* (Bill and many others refer to this as "performance-based acceptance"). By the world's standards, your worth is based on how you look, how good you are at playing the piano, how successful you are in sports, or how much money you have. It is like a game—but a very serious game—for you must win or your worth just goes out the window. If you fail to succeed, you will not be appreciated or loved in the world. After years and years of living in the world's system, it is hard for us to imagine that we are totally loved and accepted *now* because of what Christ did on the cross (and not because of what we have done and accomplished through our own efforts).

Many of us know in our *heads* that we are not able to earn our salvation, for the Bible tells us so:

> *For by grace you have been saved through faith;*
> *and that not of yourselves, it is the gift of God;*
> *not as a result of works, so that no one may boast.*
> EPHESIANS 2:8-10

When you came to the throne of grace for salvation, you realized that you had failed and fallen short of the glory of God. You humbly received what Christ has done for you on the cross. And now you want to serve and please Him. How do you do that? By performance, of course. You are intrinsically wired to try to serve God "in the flesh" (led by your emotions and your intellect), so that you will *look* a certain way, *act* a certain way, and *possess* certain things. It seems natural, doesn't it? It should seem natural, because that is the natural (default) way it works in nature and in the world.

The world's system of performance-based acceptance is based on a personal belief pattern that says, *"I must _____ in order to be acceptable to God, or myself, or others."* You can fill in the blank with whatever you want. It might be a certain level of financial prosperity. It might be trying to be that excellent Christian spouse, mother, or father. It might be a certain contour of your body. It might be a particular position of status in your school or community. It might be the behavior of your kids or employees. It might be your health. You might feel that you need to maintain a particular level of holiness or get rid of a particular sin.... The *details* really don't matter. What matters is the *belief* that "I must _____ in order to be acceptable."

This belief sets the stage for a dizzying and destructive cycle of self-effort which has a tremendously stressful impact on the human body and soul. The cycle begins with standards that are fueled by a certain level of perfection that leads to a personal sense of responsibility. This takes you down the road to bondage and inescapable failure.

*1. Standards of Acceptability: "I must live up to **this standard."***

We get drawn into the cycle of self-effort when we come to believe that we must perform at certain standards. In your soul, standards sound something like this:

"I must...
- have kids that excel in sports
- please my boss
- protect my kids
- have a good marriage
- go to church
- provide for my family
- home school my kids
- weigh less than ___ pounds
- quit looking at pornography
- have a clean house
- be loved by my spouse
- memorize scripture and pray

There are billions of possible standards. You might not be aware that they drive your life. But rest assured, you've got them, and they mean trouble. The Bible calls this "living under the Law" (Romans 3:19), a phrase which refers to the pressure and bondage we experience when we place ourselves under *any* standard that we believe will make us acceptable.

2. Perfection: "I must perform this standard **perfectly.**"

When we have standards that we feel make us acceptable to God and ourselves, they aren't an option. Failing is definitely not an option. We must meet these standards perfectly in order to have the sense of peace, fulfillment, and purpose we desire. The standard itself might not require perfection, however, whatever your standard of acceptability is, it must be met perfectly. For example, on a religious level, we might not believe that we must be totally sinless in order to be acceptable. However, we normally feel that there are *certain* sins we *must* be free from if we are to be accepted (such as addictions, adultery, swearing, R- or X-rated movies).

> When we have standards that we feel make us acceptable to God and ourselves, they aren't an option.

Whatever our standards are, if we don't keep them perfectly, we feel God's love for us is compromised. Paul described *perfection* as one of "the curses of the law" (Galatians 3:10).

3. Responsibility: "It is **my** responsibility to live up to this standard."

Something hideous begins to happen when we get to this level of the self-effort cycle. The focus changes and everything begins to get dark, lonely, and very, very heavy. When we accept the destructive sense of responsibility that says, "I must ___," chronic stress levels skyrocket. Driven by the belief that we can earn God's acceptance (and therefore gain value), we might begin to manipulate others, get angry, worry, become anxious, procrastinate, or go into denial out of fear.

My experience has been that when we decide to take responsibility to fulfill a standard on our own, God will just "let us go" and allow us to try to achieve this goal in our own strength. He will not empower us through His Spirit and we are left to our own devices and energy. These mental stressors trigger the physical stress response that quite literally eats you from the inside out. Not only is this destructive to the soul and body, but it is useless on a spiritual level (Galatians 3:3). Like so many other things that "seem right to a man," an ungodly sense of responsibility "only leads to death" (Proverbs 16:9).

*4. Bondage: "I am now **controlled** by living up to this standard!"*

If self-effort goes unchecked, it can shackle us, bind us, and put us in jail. As our thoughts become consumed with reaching our standards, the standards begin to control us (rather than us controlling them). When this happens, relationships—both with God and others—suffer terribly. Those hurt might be the neglected children of a workaholic or the ignored friends of the obsessive body-conscious athlete. Most likely, fear will also drown out the quiet voice of the Holy Spirit, quenching authentic worship and prayer. The cycle of self-effort is a trap that grabs you, ties you up, controls you, and stresses your body and soul to the max, defeating your hope for finding peace and purpose.

Let's say that one of your standards sounds like this: *I must not be overweight if I am to be acceptable.* You have been a consistent participant in Weight Watchers or Jenny Craig. You have spent a tremendous amount of time, money, and effort trying to be thin. Thoughts about what you are going to eat throughout the day consume your mind. You may have even dealt with an eating disorder earlier in your life...and fear of this problem returning haunts every day of your life. However, the harder you try the worse things get. You see yourself with disgust in front of the mirror. Instead of becoming thinner, you begin to gain weight. In frustration and failure, you give up and begin to binge on cookies, cakes, donuts, and chips

Many people on diets are motivated by guilt. This usually works for a while, but the cycle of self-effort ensures failure. As they lose weight their guilt motivation will slowly fade away. They will often go off the diet because their motivator is now gone. If they do not lose weight, or if they don't lose as much as they feel they should, they may also become discouraged and depressed and quit the diet as well. In either scenario guilt motivation does not work. By the way, it doesn't work with lust, pornography, or addictions either.

> We simply were not designed to succeed on guilt-based motivation, yet it is an inevitable consequence of the self-effort cycle.

We simply were not designed to succeed on guilt-based motivation, yet it is an inevitable consequence of the self-effort cycle. God's design is radically different: "But the goal of our instruction is love from a pure heart and a *good conscience [rather than from a guilty conscience]* and a sincere faith" (1Timothy 1:5, paraphrase mine). It works the same way with all temptations. Whether it's lying, sex, or Pop-Tarts, if you try to "just say no" in your own strength through self-effort, you make the temptations more powerful.

Scripture clearly says that sinful passions are actually *aroused* by the law (Romans 7:5). If you are living under the law in self-effort, your struggles will always be worse.

Not only does self-effort throw a wrench in our attempts to *not do* something, it is also a huge hindrance in the things we are trying *to do*. If we are trying to live through self-effort, fear of failure will distract us from our goals or cause us to procrastinate. Sometimes we might even feel paralyzed—totally unable to attempt to accomplish what we are trying to do. You don't have to look far to find examples of this type of control in your own life, do you?

Most tragically, the mental bondage caused by self-effort makes it very difficult to relate to God. It becomes an impenetrable barrier in our relationship with the Lord or others. It robs us of the unconditional love He gives and makes us hesitant to approach Him as His children. Self-effort also takes a lot of brain-power. Fear of failure takes a lot of emotional energy. Together they can drown out the still small voice of God's Spirit. We might think we are doing what He wants, but His voice may be inviting us to do something entirely different. His Word may be calling us into a place of rest. But we can't hear it. We are too busy thinking and trying to do it on our own. Controlled by the cycle of self-effort, we are consumed by trying to prove ourselves to Him, others, and ourselves.

5. Ultimate Failure: You Can't Win.

If you get sucked into the cycle of self-effort, sooner or later it's going to trap you and destroy you. You will come out as either a success or a failure—and either way, you lose.

Failure to live up to the standards is an obvious defeat. You tried; you couldn't do it. Now you have to face your fears; now you have to face your guilt. You weren't good enough, you didn't care enough, or you didn't try hard enough. You failed.

When you come full circle, you will have some new choices to make. Do you pick yourself up and try it again? If you see new hope for success you might jump back into the cycle and try it again. You might also consider "lowering the bar." Perhaps your standard was "just too high," or maybe you just need to change your definition of "acceptable." (You can usually lower your expectations for yourself, but it's unlikely that your coach, professor, parents, or boss are going to demand less of you.) And remember: When you lower the bar on the way *God* designed you to live, the natural consequences will be unavoidable (Galatians 6:7). You might be able to convince yourself that you are free to drink too much, lie, cheat, or fill your mind and body with whatever brings you pleasure, but make no mistake you will become the slave to the very things you think you are free to do. Alcoholism, prison, AIDS, and other costs await those who give in and "lower the bar."

> *What then? Shall we sin because we are not under*
> *the law but under grace? May it never be!*
> *Do you not know that when you present yourselves*
> *to someone as slaves for obedience, you are slaves*
> *of the one whom you obey, either of sin resulting in death,*
> *or obedience resulting in righteousness?*
> ROMANS 6:15-16

The cycle of self-effort can beat you up real hard; hard enough to knock the wind out of you. Then what do you do? Are you going to try again? Are you going to risk the pain of failure again? Unlikely. It's probably easier to just be known as the chubby one. It's probably safer to retreat into a life of secret sin rather than face rejection by those you respect. Perhaps you are now enduring the sneers of those who scoffed at your attempts to succeed. Perhaps you are feeling the condemnation of those who imposed their standards on you in the first place. (Your Bible study leader wags his head in distain as you share your latest struggles with lust.) Either way the fact remains: You tried and you couldn't do it. You failed.

On the other hand, let's say you come out on top a winner. You memorized your verses, you passed the exam, you dropped the pounds, or you fared well in the competition. For the moment you've faced the challenge and succeeded. You fulfilled the standard that said, "I must _____ in order to be acceptable to God, others, and myself." Well, congratulations; you are now self-righteous and full of pride. Ouch. Is that too harsh? No, not at all. Let's think about it.

When you got sucked into the cycle of self-effort you believed that, "I'll be "alright" if I do _____." Then you bought into the lie that you should do this by yourself, and then you actually did it on your own. So now that you've succeeded, you become "self-righteous" because you made yourself "right." Self-righteousness feels so good for a while, but make no mistake about it. It's a cesspool that breeds pride, arrogance, and judgment. If pride is allowed to fester, it becomes a stench—obvious to almost everyone except the person that has been swept away in its self-deception. Self-righteousness only feeds more self-effort. Success fuels the desire to jump right back into the cycle and do it all over again, and you become even *more* of a slave to the standards you have set for yourself. The self-righteous are usually brought to their senses only by graphic failure or burnout.

If you are playing the self-effort game and seem to be winning, beware. The end will come, either by force, or by choice, or by the grave. You won't be able to keep it up forever. The weight lifter's bicep will one day sag. The stock market will fall. The most upright of men slips and falls. The model's stomach will one day bulge ... and the stench of the self-righteous man's pride will be evident to all soon enough.

> **"Walking in the flesh" (Romans 8:4) defines self-effort. It emerges anytime we rely on our own intellect or emotions.**

"Walking in the flesh" (Romans 8:4) defines self-effort. It emerges anytime we rely on our own intellect or emotions. Self-effort is an attempt to gain acceptance, love, and worth by living up to certain standards in your own strength. It never brings lasting results, because the flesh is weak (Matthew 26:41), lustful (Ephesians 2:3), and polluted (Jude 23). Romans 8:8 clearly concludes that, "...those who are in the flesh cannot please God." How ironic. Your initial goal in the first place was to please God. However, your self-effort has done just the opposite.

Whether you succeed or fail, in the end you will always lose when you enter the cycle of self-effort. That's pretty disheartening stuff—but that's the bad news. The good news is this: Living by standards and self-effort was never intended to make anyone acceptable, and it was never part of God's design.

Breaking the Cycle

We've been working our tails off in a way that we were never created to work; we've been striving for a goal that we were never intended to reach. We may have accepted our salvation by grace through faith, but without a conscious renewal of our minds according to the new realities of who we are in Christ, we quickly began to serve Him by returning to our old behavior patterns—patterns of gaining our love and acceptance through our performance and our self-effort under the Law.

Please understand this: You were *designed* by God to experience stress when you try to live by self-effort! Recurring or chronic stress can be like that warning light on the dashboard of your car indicating that you are not living according to design. Self-effort doesn't work. It never did work. It won't work in the future. It doesn't work in your spirit; it doesn't work on your soul; it doesn't work for your body. Self-effort simply does not work. You don't need to try harder, you don't need to try something different, and you don't need to try again.

God designed the Law to bring us to despair and then bring us to something different. So, if you've been trying your best and still find yourself discouraged, you should be encouraged! Living under the Law and walking in the flesh through the power of self-effort have brought you precisely where God created them to bring you. They were designed to bring you to failure, and they were designed to bring you to Christ!

You were *designed* by God to experience stress when you try to live by self-effort! Recurring or chronic stress can be like that warning light on the dashboard of your car indicating that you are not living according to design.

But before faith came, we were kept in custody
under the law [in bondage to its curses]...
Therefore the Law has become our tutor to lead us to Christ,
so that we may be justified by faith.
GALATIANS 3:23-24, (paraphrase mine)

For Christ is the end of the law
for righteousness to everyone who believes.
ROMANS 10:4

He condemned sin in the flesh, so that the requirement
of the Law might be fulfilled in us, who do not walk
according to the flesh, but according to the Spirit.
For those who are according to the flesh set their minds
on the things of the flesh, but those who are according to the Spirit,
the things of the Spirit. For the mind set on the flesh is death,
but the mind set on the Spirit is life and peace,
because the mind set on the flesh is hostile toward God;
for it does not subject itself to the law of God,
for it is not even able to do so,
and those who are in the flesh cannot please God.
ROMANS 8:3

The Essential Transformation.

Yes, the world and religion have trained your intellect and your emotions to live by the flesh, in self-effort, under the law. They have done their training well, and by default, we find ourselves swept away in performance-based acceptance and the cycle of self-effort. It all began with the belief that, "I must do something in order to be accepted by God." We break that cycle by breaking this false belief and replacing it with the truth about how God loves you, unconditionally, and the truth about *who* you are, and *how* you are to live. Romans 12:2 describes the process:

And do not be conformed to this world, but be transformed
by the renewing of your mind, so that you may prove
what the will of God is, that which is good and acceptable and perfect.

Who You Are

The foundation of self-effort is shattered when we realize what is new about us, and who we have become... not because of our works, but because of what God did at the Cross and at the moment we committed our lives to Christ:

I have been crucified with Christ;
and it is no longer I who live, but Christ lives in me;
and the life which I now live in the flesh I live by faith in
the Son of God, who loved me and gave Himself up for me.
GALATIANS 2:20

Therefore if anyone is in Christ,
he is a new creature; the old things passed away;
behold, new things have come.
2 CORINTHIANS 5:17

Interesting, isn't it that many of us have devoted ourselves to attaining what God has already attained?! We try to give our lives for Jesus, but the Bible says that our old self is dead, crucified with Him. We try to get closer to Christ, but Scripture says that He actually lives within us! What lies are revealed by these truths. How this unveils one of Satan's most powerful strategies. Satan's scheme is to keep us trying harder, walking in the flesh in our own strength, according to our own inklings to become something we already are!

Walking in the flesh is wrong, even when we are trying to do "good" things such as diet, exercise, love others, or even serve God. Self-effort misses the mark; it is sin, and it defrauds God of His glory even as it destroys our lives. Paul goes so far as to say that a mind set on the flesh "is death" and "hostile toward God" (Romans 8:6-7).

The way of self-effort seems so right, but it is so wrong. We may have thought we were trying with the best of intentions, but can't you see now that those intentions are twisted and tainted? Acts of self-effort deny what is real and true and good about what God has done at the Cross, and who we are as a result. From the first moment God's Spirit came into our hearts, old things passed away, and a new way of living became a possibility.

How You Are to Live

Jesus used a powerful, yet simple illustration to communicate how we are to go about living—now that He lives in us, now that all our sin has been washed away, now that His purification has made us completely acceptable to Him:

> *I am the true vine... You are already clean because*
> *of the word which I have spoken to you. Abide in Me, and I in you.*
> *As the branch cannot bear fruit of itself unless it abides in the vine,*
> *so neither can you unless you abide in Me. I am the vine,*
> *you are the branches; he who abides in Me and I in him,*
> *he bears much fruit, for apart from Me you can do nothing.*
>
> JOHN 15:1, 3-5, (emphasis mine)

This is the truth that sets us free from the curses of the Law and the trap of self-effort. *Christ is now living through you. You can do nothing on your own. You can do all things through Him.* This new belief, then, replaces the old standards performance that said, *"I must _____ in order to be acceptable."* The new truth, in a prayer of surrender and release to God, says this, *"I can't do it! But You can! Do it, Lord!"*

This prayer is to be our repeated pledge when we face temptation and challenges big and small. It is to be our dedication at the beginning of each day, and our thanks every evening. You were designed to live in intimate unity with God, in dependence on the reality of His Spirit in yours, moment by moment, hour after hour, until that day when, through the death of your fleshly body, your unity becomes complete.

The Motivation of the Heart

It all boils down to the motivation of the heart. Your motivation will be revealed by your level of stress and finding the answers to some honest questions: Why am I doing the things that I am doing? Why am I behaving the way I am behaving? Am I trying to gain approval and acceptance? If the answers uncover self-effort, nothing can result except failure or self-righteousness as you are again caught up under the burden and yoke of the law. However, if the motivation of your heart is to be dominated by the Spirit and surrender to the will of God, then you will not carry out the deeds of the flesh, but instead, you will be walking in the Spirit. Learning and understanding the core motivation for our actions makes the critical difference. The question that reveals our motivation is always the same: Am I seeking value and worth by my actions? Or am I believing God for what He has said and then acting by faith upon it?

A believer who is dominated by the Spirit will seek God's truth in His Word with the sole purpose of activating their will to line up with that truth— no matter what the intellect or feelings are saying or doing. Just hearing God's truth does absolutely nothing for the believer. God's Word too must become a matter of the heart, as we remember *who* we are and *how* we are to live. The power of the Word is unleashed when we choose to allow the Spirit within us to act on those truths:

> *But prove yourselves doers of the word, and not merely hearers*
> *who delude themselves. For if anyone is a hearer of the word and not a doer,*
> *he is like a man who looks at his natural face in a mirror;*
> *for once he has looked at himself and gone away, he has immediately*
> *forgotten what kind of person he was. But one who looks intently*
> *at the perfect law, the law of liberty, and abides by it,*
> *not having become a forgetful hearer but an effectual doer,*
> *this man will be blessed in what he does.*
> JAMES 1:22-25

A Christian who is abiding in Christ and walking in the Spirit is dominated by the Spirit of God that is now living within them. Their motivation is based on knowing that they are loved by God unconditionally and have been reconciled to God by no work of their own. Bill calls this "love motivation." Because of their love for God, they begin renewing their mind with God's truth under the guidance of the Holy Spirit that now indwells their spirit. The apostle Paul summarized this motivation from the heart in 2 Corinthians 5:14-15:

> For the love of Christ controls us ...
> so that they who live might no longer live for themselves,
> but for Him who died and rose again on their behalf.

This motivation of love will be in continual tension with the flesh and the law. The temptation to return to self-effort will always be with us. Satan and the world, of course, will always attempt to draw us back into self-effort.

> But I say, walk by the Spirit, and you will not carry out the desire
> of the flesh. For the flesh sets its desire against the Spirit,
> and the Spirit against the flesh; for these are in opposition to one another,
> so that you may not do the things that you please.
> But if you are led by the Spirit, you are not under the Law.
> GALATIANS 5:16-18

> But the fruit of the Spirit is love, joy, peace, patience,
> kindness, goodness, faithfulness, gentleness, self-control;
> against such things there is no law. Now those who belong to
> Christ Jesus have crucified the flesh with its passions and desires.
> GALATIANS 5:22-24

Let me ask another question: What law could be written that would make you display peace in your life? Or for that matter faithfulness, gentleness, and self-control? I certainly cannot think of one. Scripture clearly points out that there is no law that can create these qualities in your life. These qualities become evident within your life only by abiding in Christ, walking in the Spirit, humbling yourself, and then aligning your will with God's will.

Walking in the Spirit—in complete dependence and submission to the Spirit of Christ in you—shatters the cycle of self-effort and unleashes the power of God. You are no longer responsible for the results. The results are left to God, and He gets the glory for what He does. Stress, fear, and anxiety

When you abide in Christ and walk in the Spirit, you are connected *directly* to the power source, the Lord...not wearing down your own batteries through self-effort.

give way to healing—not only in your soul, but also in your body as well. Instead of being continually exhausted and worn down, personal energy is continually renewed. When you abide in Christ and walk in the Spirit, you are connected *directly* to the power source, the Lord...not wearing down your own batteries through self-effort. Because chronic stress is relieved, the immune system strengthens and all of the body's natural defenses improve.

Yet those who wait for the LORD will gain new strength; they will mount up with wings like eagles, they will run and not get tired, they will walk and not become weary.
ISAIAH 40:31

Humility and Humbleness before God

Abiding in Christ and breaking the cycle of self-effort requires that you humble yourself before God. God needs to be God and man must realize that he is man. In other words, we need to put God where God belongs (in control) and man needs to be placed where man belongs (worshiping at the feet of God). While this is freeing, it is not easy. In order to be free from stress, we must abandon our attempts to be like God, who alone controls the world and those around us. That's tough, requiring that we bow our knee to Him in submission, recognize Him as the sovereign Lord of all, and repent of our fleshly desires to be like Him in these respects. Recognizing that we have been crucified with Him and that He now lives in us is a *continual* process marked by a first time decision to surrender all we have, and all we are, and all we do.

Humble yourselves under the mighty hand of God, that He might exalt you at the proper time, casting all your anxiety upon Him, because He cares for you.
1 PETER 5:6-7

Surrendering your will to the obedience of Christ through the Holy Spirit that now dwells in you allows an alignment of your will with God's will. As a result, obedience now comes naturally (or should I say "supernaturally"). The bondage of the world's system is broken, setting you free from the destructive power of the law and the stress amplifying consequences of self-effort.

By abiding in Christ and allowing Him to live His life through you, you reclaim His original design for intimacy and oneness. Now when you read God's Word and His truth is illuminated, you can choose to align your will with His written desires and the leading of His Spirit in you regardless of what your emotions or intellect are telling you.

A great illustration of this can be found in the movie *First Knight,* a story about King Arthur, Lady Guinevere, and Sir Lancelot in Camelot. As the tale of commitment, love, and tragedy opens, Lady Guinevere has made a decision to marry King Arthur and become his queen. Throughout the trials and conflicts of the land she encounters Sir Lancelot, a young and dashing knight. Sir Lancelot has committed his will to serving King Arthur, the Knights of the Round Table, and Camelot. Yet after twice rescuing Lady Guinevere and several chance meetings, affection begins to stir in Sir Lancelot, affections that Lady Guinevere feels toward him as well. The plot thickens as they struggle with these intense feelings, while trying to remain true to the commitments they had previously made to their king.

After deep soul searching, Sir Lancelot decides that the best way he can be true to the commitment he has made to King Arthur and Camelot is to leave. But as he goes to tell Lady Guinevere of his decision, they are caught up in a passionate moment and a kiss, which is interrupted unexpectedly by King Arthur.

King Arthur later confronts Lady Guinevere and asks her if she loves Sir Lancelot. She replies that she does. He questions her further and asks if she loves him. She states very forcefully that she does. King Arthur in frustration asks, "How can you love two men?" She says that there are different faces of love and she chooses to love him and him alone. King Arthur says, "You love me with your will, however, you love Sir Lancelot with your heart." Guinevere quickly responds by saying, "Well, you have the best of it, because my will is stronger than my heart. Do you think that I put such a high price on my feelings? Feelings last for a moment but my will holds me steady for my course through life."

Sir Lancelot was loyal to King Arthur and felt that the best way to remain true to this commitment was to not listen to the emotions of love and passion swelling within him and instead activate his will to leave. Certainly Guinevere, by an act of her will, was faithful to King Arthur. A moment of strong emotion revealed the feelings of each (a mistake with grave implications) but in the end, the strength of their wills prevailed as both of them repented and acted on what they knew was true and right: *Love from the will endures.*

Isn't that the way the life of a Christian should be? While the rest of the world is swept away by intellect and emotion, we (as a choice of our will) respond to His love with our love, surrendering our will to our King. Yet remember, even this choice is not something that we were designed to make in self-effort. It can be done only in His strength as His Spirit moves within ours. Our position is one of rest and of surrender. He is the One who makes it happen. That is the target to aim for, and that is the life that Jesus, in His perfection, modeled for us.

He is the one who said, "I can do nothing on My own initiative ... I do not seek My own will, but the will of Him who sent Me" (John 5:30). The motivation of Christ's heart was most evident in the Garden of Gethsemane. There, on His knees before His father, He asked that "if possible" the way of the Cross might be avoided. But His will and His love for the Father and for us prevailed as Jesus concluded His prayer with these words to the Father: "Your will be done" (Matthew 26:36-42).

Yes, it all boils down to the motivation of the heart. Are you trying to please God by your own self-effort? Or have you humbled yourself to the point that you have surrendered your will to God's Word and the Spirit of God that now dwells in you, relying on His strength alone to do the things He asks? Only you know the answers to those questions. Only you can, in humility and submission, repent of self-effort and utter the heart-felt prayer, *"I can't, but You can. Please do it, Lord."*

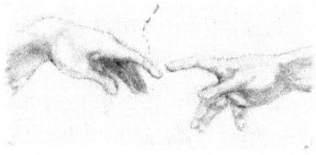

CHAPTER 4

Unresolved Anger

Do not let the sun go down on your anger,

and do not give the devil an opportunity.

EPHESIANS 4:26-27

Part 1—UNRESOLVED ANGER

When Karen came in to my office, the pain on her face was obvious. Deep creases of stress on her forehead gave way to dark and sunken eyes—eyes that flitted this way and that, never making contact with mine. With both embarrassment and desperation in her voice, she began to describe her symptoms: lack of energy, continual tiredness, erratic sleep patterns, feelings of hopelessness... She appeared to be suffering from classic depression, yet it didn't make sense considering her circumstances. Karen was attractive, married to a loving Christian police officer, and had a successful career of her own. Together they lived a life of freedom and adventure, driving nice cars and traveling the globe.

Most concerning to me, however, were her disjointed thoughts. Unable to focus and concentrate, Karen could no longer navigate through the tasks of a normal day, her mind recoiling in a dark fog of confusion and emotion. After talking a bit more, I prescribed an antidepressant, and strongly encouraged her to make an appointment with Bill at Christian Life Ministries.

Bill had a waiting list of three weeks, which was enough time for the antidepressants to begin to stabilize Karen's thoughts and emotions. When Karen and her husband, Richard, met with Bill, they began to search for the roots of her depression. After some probing, Karen began to describe a strong desire to have kids. Yet deep debt had shackled them to a dual income, and Karen had always wanted to be a stay-at-home mom. Several months ago, there had been hope on the horizon. Richard was due for a promotion, but had been passed by. She looked briefly at Richard and broke down in tears before she could finish the story.

After an awkward silence, Richard began to complete the story, and as he did his jaw began to tighten, his fists clenched, and his voice began to shake. He was an excellent police officer and in the last years had gone far above and beyond his required duties to serve the department and the community. As a plainclothes detective, he had a stellar record and was considered by everyone to be a shoo-in for the promotion to sergeant. But only a week before the decision was made, Richard left one of his shifts 15 minutes early to have a beer with some friends. Another officer noticed this infraction (purchase and consumption of alcohol while on duty), and reported it to the chief. When the dust settled, he had been passed up for the promotion and given a reprimand. The sergeant's position went to the officer who had reported him to the chief.

At this point Richard's emotions erupted into shouts and accusations against the chief and the officer. Then he turned his frustration toward Karen, who had been continually berating him for destroying his career over a single drink. He resented her cut downs, was frustrated by her withdrawal during this difficult time, and felt rejected by her refusals for physical intimacy. Finally, Richard turned his anger on himself. Before Bill and Karen, he chastised himself for his stupidity, and wept over the way it had destroyed their plans.

Anger. The dictionary defines it with synonyms such as "hostility, indignation, exasperation, pain, and affliction." (Interestingly, in British English, the root of the word "anger" also refers to "inflammation" or "a sore.") In ear-

lier chapters, I revealed the tremendous health consequences of excessive, prolonged stress, and described
many of the common circumstances that can cause it. Of
all the things that cause stress, anger is one of the most
powerful and pervasive. Bill feels that one of the greatest
sources of physical and mental illness in the world today
is unresolved anger. It is one of the first things he explores
with his clients, and in over 25 years of counseling, Bill can recall only a
handful of situations where unresolved anger was not a significant issue.

...one of the greatest
sources of physical
and mental illness in
the world today is
unresolved anger.

Much of the time anger is displayed through "getting mad." But just as
often, an angry person may not appear mad at all. Oftentimes the anger is
turned inward and the person displays hurt, offended feelings, withdrawal, or
passiveness. Anger turned inward sometimes finds its expression in self-muti-
lation and self-defeating behaviors. Sometimes anger pushes one into the
depths of depression. In the worst of situations, anger that is not dealt with
can bring a person to the point of suicide or murder.

Anger in and of itself is not a sin. Jesus became angry when he entered
the temple and saw the moneychangers defiling the place of worship. He
turned over tables, chased the merchants out with a whip, and shouted, "It
is written, 'My house shall be called a house of prayer;' but you are making
it a robbers' den!" (Matthew 21:13). Numerous examples in the Old
Testament speak of God's anger being kindled against Israel's disobedience
and other unrighteousness.

"Be angry, and yet do not sin," Ephesians 4:26 instructs us (showing that
anger can *lead* to sin, yet is not inherently sinful). Yet this passage also warns
us very clearly to "not let the sun go down on your anger." When anger is not
dealt with as God designed, the angry person can descend into a dangerous,
destructive pit that leads to relational, emotional, and even physical death.

One of the results of unresolved anger may be bitterness (Hebrews
12:14-15) and resentment. Anger often leads to vengeance. A vindictive
heart can express itself in many ways, but its intent is always the same: to
hurt the person who has hurt us. It might show up through calculated rumors
or gossip, an intentional severing of the relationship, or simply giving the
silent treatment. Anger that is not resolved does not dissipate with time. It
only festers, consuming the "victim," often imprisoning them in the bondage
of ungratefulness and hatred. In time, anger leads to a loss of hope, and a
weakened faith.

Most of us feel that our anger hurts the individual toward whom we are angry. I personally believe that this is the main reason why most of us have so much difficulty dealing with anger properly. Our emotions and our intellect *want* to hurt that individual, as least as much as they hurt us, perhaps even more. Scripture clearly shows us that unresolved anger primarily hurts *us*. Anger that is not resolved properly has many consequences to our soul and our body. (The consequences are listed in Table 1) You may experience all of these consequences or may experience only a few. However, unresolved anger can eventually lead to depression and possibly even death.

TABLE 1
Potential Consequences of Unresolved Anger
Hurt and Anger
Bitterness (Hebrews 12:14-15)
Resentment (James 3:14-16)
Vengeance (Proverbs 24:29)
Hatred (Galatians 5:20)
Ungratefulness (Romans 1:21)
Loss of Hope and Faith
Depression
Death

The Physical Effects of Unresolved Anger

The mind/body connection is very evident when you investigate the physical and health consequences of unresolved anger. Unresolved anger causes intense stress on the body. It kicks the stress response into high gear and keeps it going full throttle, loading up the body with high levels of adrenaline, cortisol, and free radicals. This, of course, increases oxidative stress and inflammation to unnatural levels, leading to premature aging and chronic degenerative disease.

Anger also causes a significant depletion in our neurotransmitters. Neurotransmitters are special biochemicals that the brain uses to send messages to other parts of the body. Important neurotransmitters include serotonin, dopamine, and norepinephrine. Persistent feelings and

Unresolved anger causes intense stress on the body.

thoughts of anger cause the body to use these important neurotransmitters at an unnatural rate and they soon become depleted. Strong feelings of hopelessness and depression will soon follow. (Depressed individuals often consider suicide, and each year 30,000 people in the U.S. alone will follow through with those thoughts.) By the time my patients become clinically depressed, they do not even relate their depression to any unresolved anger or bitterness.

Physicians normally treat the *symptoms* of depression with medication. Antidepressants primarily work by increasing the amount of selected neurotransmitters. When these neurotransmitters have increased, the symptoms of depression are improved. The use of antidepressant medication has skyrocketed over the past decade. What is so concerning is the fact that once a patient starts these antidepressants, many never seem to be able to come off them or must return to taking them once they quit. The drugs help relieve the symptoms of depression, but they can't deal with the underlying *cause* of the majority of cases of depression: unresolved anger. This is why Bill and the counselors at Christian Life Ministries focus and spend so much time searching for those areas of anger that the client has not dealt with properly. If this anger is not dealt with, the success of their counseling is very limited and usually of no lasting value.

As a physician, I still prescribe antidepressant medication for depression because I have learned that the antidepressants are able to give my patients a quicker response, but it is a limited response unless they deal with the issues of the soul that are causing the physical symptoms. I often encourage my Christian patients to consider biblical counseling so they can deal with the cause, and not just the symptoms of their depression. If they combine biblical counseling with their medication, they not only are able to resolve their depression but also they are often able to get off their medication and remain off their medication permanently.

Sources of Anger

The world is not a happy place. Since the "fall of man" in the Garden of Eden, life has been a constant dance with disappointment, emptiness, and pain. Relationships turn sour. Friends turn their backs. Family members wound us in our most vulnerable spots. Others unknowingly hurt us, leaving us with wounds that scar. Through it all, anger becomes a regular companion, emerging anytime that something we want to happen doesn't (or something that we don't want to happen does happen.) Whenever we can't get to something that we feel is essential to a meaningful, secure, fulfilled life, we will get angry at whatever is standing in the way.

Broken Expectations

Anger is fueled by the breaking of hopeful expectations—whether it's broken eggs or broken promises. We all have certain expectations about how life should "work out" and we have expectations about how those we love and care about should act toward us. If your spouse tells you that they will be home at 6:00 p.m. for dinner and then shows up at 8:30 p.m. without calling, you would become angry especially if that violated a strong expectation and was a reflection of something that was important to you, such as trust or respect. This is one of the areas that is very important to my wife. I try not to ever be late. If I get stuck in an emergency at the hospital or an unexpected delivery, I've learned to give her a call. She expects it and being sensitive to that expectation is one of the ways I can show her love and respect.

Expectations can also be nonverbal. Each of us has assumptions about life that we think are universal and shared by everyone. That's not always the case, and our expectations are normally much higher for those we are close to. When people do not act in the way you expect them to act, it can hurt you deeply and create a tremendous amount of anger. This is why we seem to be hurt more by those who love us than we are by strangers. Haven't you caught yourself telling a loved one that if they would only treat you like they would treat a total stranger you would be thrilled? Oftentimes loved ones *do* treat casual acquaintances with much more kindness and respect than they do us—but be honest, you do the same thing! Still, it causes plenty of anger as heartfelt expectations are broken.

Blocked Desires

Closely related to broken expectations are blocked desires. A "desire" is a wish; it's a hope for something that you really want (or don't want). You don't necessarily expect it to happen, but you are pretty convinced that life would be better if it did. The problem is that desires are not under your control. In order for a desire to be fulfilled, you must have the cooperation of someone else. For example, you might desire a healthy, vibrant marriage. The problem is that it takes two to make that happen, and your spouse might not share that desire or might not have the ability to do his or her part.

A "goal," on the other hand, is an objective that is under your control. Unlike a desire, which is dependent on others, a goal is something that can be reached with the resources you have available. For example, a reasonable goal would be to say, "I want to be a strong, accepting spouse to my mate." Nothing can stop you from doing that as long as you do it in the Spirit and not through self-effort.

Anger is inevitable if you don't view desires and goals differently. If you have spent any time watching *American Idol,* you quickly see what I mean. The participants have made it their goal to win. (However, this really isn't a goal; it's a desire, because it can be blocked by the panel of three judges.) The cameras catch them leaving their audition and generally many of their comments are met with bleeps to cancel out what they are saying in their anger. The show's popularity is based heavily on the fact that many of these participants have unrealistic desires, and when they are blocked it abruptly creates a tremendous amount of anger.

In your case, you might desire your children or spouse act in a certain way, and that's fine. But remember, except for using handcuffs and straitjackets, you can't control them anymore than they can control you. Always remember, a desire *is something that you wish would happen, but is ultimately out of your control.* A goal *is something that you can control.* If you don't have all the resources to make something happen, it's not a goal; it's a desire. If you get them mixed up, you will get angry when circumstances beyond your control interfere.

Do you want a very quick hint for radically reducing anger and stress in your life? Apply these two strategies:

1. *Pray for your desires.* God commands you to do this anyway (Matthew 6:9-13; John 16:24). You might desire that your children turn out to be honest, respectful, obedient teens. But that's not in your control, as any parent of a teen can tell you. Pray for them!

2. *Act on your goals.* In the case of parenting teens, don't try to change them; instead, make it your goal to be a solid, gracious, guiding mom or dad—regardless of what *they* do. You can control only what you do, so act! Sure, you may have to ground them and provide firm barriers, but everyone will be a lot less angry (including you) if you are doing it out of a loving, serving heart—rather than out of anger because they aren't doing what you want.

Part 2: THE FORGIVENESS FACTOR

Healing in the Design

Anger is a given in a fallen world. Whether it is expressed with violent outbursts or in solemn silence, once anger has raised its head it is critical that it is dealt with properly. The reason is very clear: Unresolved anger can destroy the body and soul, just as it has the potential of destroying the core of your being and your relationship with the Lord and others. Thankfully, God has not left us without clear instruction and the resources to deal with it.

God is the Great Physician (Exodus 15:26). He embodies the true heart of a dedicated doctor. He is intimately acquainted with how we are made, for indeed, we are the work of His hands (Psalm 139). He is the Wonderful Counselor (Isaiah 9:6), knowing the intricate and integrated nature of our souls and our spirits. Like no one else, God is the One most qualified to prescribe a remedy for our pain and heal the destruction caused by our anger. As our Great Provider (Genesis 22:14), God not only offers His instruction, but also He Himself has intervened and provided a strategic way out of the bondage of anger. *It's the way of forgiveness,* the way that He Himself walked as He carried the cross to that hill outside of Jerusalem—and it's the way that He now beckons us to follow.

> He Himself has intervened and provided a strategic way out of the bondage of anger. It's the way of forgiveness...

Forgiveness is the divine transaction, paid in full by the blood of Jesus, which frees both the offender and the offended from the bondage of sin. The act of forgiveness follows in the footsteps of Christ to the very shadows of the cross, where healing, liberty, and power find their genesis in His punishment and death.

Contrary to earthly wisdom and human conceptions of "fairness," true biblical forgiveness is built on the following principles:

First, forgiveness is built on the understanding that all sin is ultimately against God, not us. David recognized this fact when he repented of his sins of adultery and murder. He proclaimed, "Against You, You only, I have sinned" (Psalm 51:4). It certainly seems like others sin against us, but remember, we are no longer our own (Romans 14:7-8). *We belong to Him.* He is the true owner of all that we are, and any attack against us is an attack against Him. When Paul was pursuing the destruction of Christians, Jesus blinded him, knocked him from his donkey, and bellowed, "Saul, Saul, why are you persecuting *Me?*" (Acts 9:4) When others persecute you, they are really persecuting Jesus through you as well.

As members of the greater church of God, we are members of His body (1 Corinthians 12:27). Each of us occupies a specific part in that body, but we are only a *part* of the whole; the "whole" is Jesus. An offense against one part is an offense against the entire body. This is understood in the words we commonly use to describe an attack. If "Kevin" gets stabbed in the back, the newspapers don't say, "A back was stabbed yesterday." They say, "Kevin was stabbed in the back." Likewise, you might function as an arm in the body of Christ. When you get stabbed, however, the offense is against Jesus, who is the entire body. The wound that He received came through you.

The fact that all sin is against God is an extension of this spiritual reality: We no longer live, but Christ is the one who lives in us (Galatians 2:20). So when someone sins against you, it's still going to hurt. They even may have meant to hurt you; but you are His now, and the sin is against Him. In this way "we share the sufferings of Christ." (I Peter 4:12-13). Paul described it this way:

Now I rejoice in my sufferings for your sake,
and in my flesh I do my share on behalf of His body,
which is the church, in filling up what is lacking in Christ's afflictions.
COLOSSIANS 1:24

This may seem odd, but it is a vital truth to grasp. When we understand that we are part of Him, we are able to bring the process of forgiveness all the way to the Cross—where forgiveness is completed. If we think the sin is ultimately against us, we will be left to deal with it in our own strength and wisdom—and we were never designed to do that. Forgiveness finds its origin at the cross when we accept the fact that the sin was actually against Him and dealt with by Him. The sin was a blow by another striking the part of Christ's body that happens to be us. In the space of time, the sin is just occurring, so the pain and anger are just being felt. Thus, we "share in His suffering." It's an extension of the fact we were truly crucified with Christ (Galatians 2:20).

Second, true forgiveness is empowered when we embrace the extent of God's forgiveness toward us. Those who feel they have been forgiven of little, forgive little; those who know that they have been forgiven of much, forgive much (Luke 7:47). Psalm 103:3-4 says that the Lord "pardons all your iniquities" and "redeems your life from the pit...." Paul expresses God's forgiveness with these words:

> *In Him we have redemption through His blood,*
> *the forgiveness of our trespasses, according to the riches*
> *of His grace which He lavished on us.*
> EPHESIANS 1:7-8

> *He made you alive together with Him,*
> *having forgiven us all our transgressions,*
> *having canceled out the certificate of debt consisting*
> *of decrees against us, which was hostile to us;*
> *and He has taken it out of the way, having nailed it to the cross.*
> COLOSSIANS 2:13-14

Note that these passages are all in the past tense. God's forgiveness was perfectly paid two thousand years ago. In order for us to authentically extend forgiveness to others, we must first realize that we have been forgiven. Understanding the incredible extent of God's forgiveness for us gives us a perspective from which we can extend forgiveness to others, no matter how bad their actions seem. When we forgive, we are just passing on something that we already have from Him, something that he freely gave us in infinitely greater measure. In that way, we forgive, "just as the Lord forgave you" (Colossians 3:13).

Understanding the incredible extent of God's forgiveness for us gives us a perspective from which we can extend forgiveness to others, no matter how bad their actions seem.

Third, in order to be willing to forgive, we must first trust God with our feelings. Forgiveness is an act of the will, not the emotions or intellect. Satan and the world have caused us to get this backward. Most people don't forgive because they don't feel like it. If you follow your feelings, you'll never truly forgive, for your anger will always get in the way. If you trust God with those feelings, however, and choose to obey God's call to forgive, the peace will follow *after* you forgive.

Fourth, forgiveness is something that God must do through us; it's not something we can do on our own (John 15:5). Therefore, forgiving is impossible to truly do through self-effort. True and lasting forgiveness must be done as a choice of your will as you align your will with His. Your will, not your emotions, must lead the way as you walk toward forgiveness in the power of the Spirit. Even if you understand how to forgive, you must realize that only He can do it... and actually, *it has already been done.* Just as Christ's death on the cross is "past tense" and all our sins have been forgiven, the fact that we have been crucified with Him also means that the ultimate price of sins against us by others has been paid for when we were crucified with Him. We simply have the privilege of passing on that payment.

Just as we were the part of the body stricken by the blow of another's sin, we are the part of the body through which God's completed forgiveness is passed. We actually get to participate in the power of God's love as it is extended through us and forgive those who have sinned against Christ through us! He actually uses us as a conduit for His forgiveness.

Reasons We Don't Forgive

Forgiveness brings healing and freedom to the person who has been offended and releases the destructive stress that unresolved anger causes. So why is it so hard? Why are we so hesitant? Here are some of the excuses you might use to dodge God's command to forgive:

- The sin was "too bad" and hurt "too much."
- They aren't sorry.
- They may do it again.
- I don't like them.
- They haven't asked me to forgive them.
- They did it on purpose.
- I can't forget it.
- I'll have to treat them better.
- I want to punish them.

You can hide behind any one of those excuses if you want to, but don't kid yourself. If you choose not to forgive, the consequences are grave.

Consequences of unforgiveness:

- A restriction of love, even toward those who did not cause the pain
- Fear of being vulnerable
- Stress and all its effects (e.g., increased free radicals, depleted immune system, ulcers, and maybe even a chronic degenerative disease)
- Inability to "get over it," resulting in bondage to the hurtful event or person

- "Opportunity" is given to Satan (Ephesians 4:27)
- "Advantage" is given to Satan (2 Corinthians 2:10-11)
- Being handed over to "the tormenter" (Matthew 18:23-35)
- Depression and even possibly death
- A hindered relationship with God (Isaiah 59:2)

Steps to Forgiveness

Forgiving by self-effort is impossible. Forgiveness was initiated by God, embodied in Christ's blood, and is empowered through the Holy Spirit. If you need to forgive, begin by asking God to work through you entirely, giving you the willingness and the ability to walk through the process.

1. Make a list of the specific hurts that were committed against you. List both the things they did and didn't do that hurt you.

2. List all the ways this action has affected you. (Your pain will help guide you to the consequences of the person's offense against you.) For example, if someone steals your car, you might be mad because you have to work overtime to buy a new one. If your spouse has left you, you might be depressed because of how it has caused other couples to feel awkward around you or avoid you. The personal ramifications of another's sin against you might be financial, social, mental, emotional, physical, or others.

3. Claim the truth that your life is Christ's. As part of His body, you shared in His suffering. Thank God for His forgiveness *toward* you, and thank Him for forgiving the offender through you. Pass the sin on to the Cross. Since God has already paid the price for this offense, pass God's forgiveness on to the offender.

4. Release the responsibility for punishment to God. While you may still need to pursue legal recourse or church discipline, recognize that it is not your place to punish. Forgiveness doesn't mean you have to forget, however. If someone has sinned against you, you don't have to be foolish and set yourself up for further pain or abuse. It does mean, however, that in God's power, you free them from your condemnation and judgment, and choose to love them...faults and all. "'Vengeance is Mine...,' says the Lord" (Romans 12:19).

A prayer of forgiveness might sound something like this:

Father of Forgiveness,

Oh, Lord, you are aware of the sins that have been committed and the effect they have had on me as Your child. (Give Him the specifics.) I know that my life is Your life and all I am and all I do is through You. So, thank You for forgiving them through me. Thanks for paying the cost for their sin and mine when You died on the cross and when I was crucified with You. I trust in You to punish them as You see fit. I choose not to do that in anyway on my own. Free me from my feelings of anger. Make me a blessing to those that have hurt me.

Your forgiven child.

5. Destroy the lists you made from items 1 and 2 above. Destroying the lists symbolizes that you are no longer choosing to carry the burden of their sin. You are letting it go; you are setting yourself free!

6. Give a blessing. A caring act of kindness in the face of an offense seems to be the fuel that unleashes the supernatural power of forgiveness and breaks the stronghold of emotion that Satan uses to control those who have been hurt. Proverbs 21:14 says that, "A gift in secret subdues anger." First Peter 3:8-9 commands us to respond this way:

> *To sum up, all of you be harmonious, sympathetic,*
> *brotherly, kindhearted, and humble in spirit;*
> *not returning evil for evil or insult for insult,*
> *but giving a blessing instead.*

I know that's not "fair." I know they don't "deserve it." But some sort of blessing given to the offender is great for your body and soul. You really have to experience this to understand it. But I am telling you that giving some sort of "good" to those who have done you wrong is cleansing and liberating! It is so contrary to the ways of the world and the flesh. It will destroy any lingering attachment you have to anger and frustration and will be the final act that sets you free from the sin that another has committed against you and Christ.

Those are the steps to genuine and lasting forgiveness. Before we continue on, looking at two other critical aspects of forgiveness, I want to encourage you to stop here, let this soak in for a while, and pray for God's leading in what He now wants to do through you. Forgiving others is so vital to every aspect of our being.... Please don't just hear about it without pausing to let God unleash its healing and restoring power.

Father,

Search my heart and show me Your ways. As my Redeemer, I praise You for forgiving me. Be now my courage, showing me

*specific areas where I have been hurt. Align my will with Your's,
make me willing to be a channel of Your forgiving love to those
who have harmed me, then do it for Your name's sake!
Amen.*

The Hardest One to Forgive

Reconciliation with God is absolutely central to finding health and peace in this life and the one to come. Forgiveness also sets the stage for healing and restoration in earthly relationships. Time and time again, people are set free as they begin to forgive each other. Accepting the forgiveness of God through Christ is where it all begins. We are then to extend forgiveness to those around us, resulting in freedom and health for our souls and bodies.

But that leaves one relationship left to deal with—and for many reasons, this is sometimes the hardest person to forgive. How is it that you can receive God's forgiveness, forgive others, and yet not be willing to forgive *yourself?* Forgiving yourself for the sins you commit is an important step of obedience, and it can be very, very difficult. There are several possible reasons for this:

- *You don't feel forgiven.* Guilt runs deep and Satan loves to stir it up. While we might feel forgiven for some sins, there are others that our emotions seem to be unable to let go. Usually these are "big" sins that we feel are unpardonable, or "lesser" sins that have had great impact. (I know it's easier to forgive yourself for cheating on a spelling test than it is to believe you are forgiven for your abortion or your affair.) In these situations, we feel we've gone too far to be forgiven. Our *feelings* of guilt condemn us over and over until our minds believe that we really aren't forgiven at all.

- *You hold yourself to higher standards than God does.* Even though you believe that God has forgiven you for certain sins, it's quite possible that you choose not to forgive yourself for them. This reveals that your standards for acceptability are higher than God's and, again, reveals a vein of self-effort and a desire to be your own god. Think about this logically: If a perfectly holy God now finds you completely acceptable because of the Cross, who are you to demand more of yourself? (See Romans 8:1).

- *You think you need to punish yourself.* Self-punishment comes from thoughts that say, *I must pay for my own sins. Christ didn't do the job well enough, so I need to punish myself before I can be forgiven.*

Self-punishment might make you feel better for a moment, but it never lasts, and leads to intensified self-destructive behavior.

- *You know your motives.* It can be easier to forgive someone when we think that maybe they didn't mean to do it. But when it comes to dealing with ourselves, often we know the bitter truth: Most of our sins come from conscious choices to do wrong. Knowing our motives also makes us fearful that we will probably commit them again if we are in the same circumstances and might make us question the sincerity of our repentance.

When You Don't Forgive Yourself

God has chosen to fully forgive you, but you are the one that must choose to forgive yourself. If you choose not to, and continue to live in the lie, some weighty consequences await you:

- *A life of heavy burdens.* Thoughts of guilt and shame are a huge load upon anyone, and the weight of it is something we were never designed to carry. Christ took that weight upon Himself and now offers a different kind of load for us to carry:

> *"Come to Me, all who are weary and heavy-laden,*
> *and I will give you rest. Take My yoke upon you and learn from Me,*
> *for I am gentle and humble in heart, and you will find rest for your souls.*
> *For My yoke is easy and My burden is light."*
> MATTHEW 11:28-30

- *Self Punishment.* This one hurts, sometimes literally. Unless we forgive ourselves, we will always be prone to beating ourselves up emotionally, denying ourselves good things that God offers, and sometimes even hurting ourselves physically...maybe even to the point of suicide. You can choose to continue to condemn yourself if you want to, but know that God doesn't. Your choice to punish yourself is in direct contradiction to what the Bible says is true:

> *Therefore there is now no condemnation for those*
> *who are in Christ Jesus. For the law of the Spirit of life in*
> *Christ Jesus has set you free from the law of sin and death.*
> ROMANS 8:1-2

- *Feelings of Unworthiness.* Satan rejoices when we feel as if our sin has disqualified us from the Master's service and made us useless to His Kingdom. The truth is that God has *always* been in the business of using dented people for His glory. Numerous people in the Bible had to fall hard before they were willing to give up their self-effort and let God begin to live through them. Moses, David, Paul, Peter and many others failed miserably ... and yet they were used mightily for God's glory.

> *For we are His workmanship, created in Christ Jesus*
> *for good works, which God prepared beforehand*
> *so that we would walk in them.*
> EPHESIANS 2:10

- *Excessive Self-Effort.* If we don't forgive ourselves, we may begin to try even harder to make things right. We think that, *If I just do such and such, I'll feel better about myself.* Certainly, earthly consequences of our sin might require quite a bit of effort to fix (if they can be fixed at all), but if we set out to make ourselves feel acceptable before God, we have missed the mark again and launch ourselves right back into self-effort ... the very thing that got us in trouble in the first place.

> *For the one who has entered His rest has himself*
> *also rested from his works, as God did from His.*
> *Therefore let us be diligent to enter that rest,*
> *so that no one will fall...*
> HEBREWS 4:10-11

- *Damage to Your Body.* If you are unwilling to forgive yourself, a tremendous amount of anger is turned inward, against yourself, causing significant mental and physical stress, resulting in all the damage we have described previously.
  When I kept silent about my sin, my body wasted away....
  My vitality was drained away as with the fever heat of summer.
> PSALM 32:3-4

- *A victim mentality.* Unforgiveness of self can result in a pitiful display of false humility. Leave self-flagellation in the dark ages. It's a pathetic way to draw attention to yourself and it's a disgraceful way to manipulate the sympathy of others.

When we refuse to extend forgiveness to ourselves, we are ultimately choosing to disobey and place our ways above God's. This *mis*aligns your will and His, and makes an abiding relationship with Him a farce. If you don't forgive yourself, you're saying that you have standards that are higher than His. You're saying that you are unwilling to trust in His strength to do what He commands. It's not just bad for you; it's wrong.

Letting Go

If you've been holding on to a past sin, I don't have to tell you what it's like, do I? You are probably dealing with at least one, if not several of the consequences of unforgiveness.

The truth is, God has done His part and our forgiveness is fully granted from Him. But total reconciliation requires *both* parties to forgive. God has forgiven. Are you willing to allow Him to show you how to forgive yourself? In order to proceed according to God's design, you must be willing to let Him into those dark areas of your life so He can give you the desire and the power to forgive yourself too. What would Paul's life and ministry have been like if he was unwilling to forgive himself for actually killing Christians before his conversion? After looking at Paul's ministry and life, I would have to conclude that he was certainly able to forgive himself and relish the love and freedom that comes with God's forgiveness.

If you have reached the point where you know that God is telling you that it's time to let go, that it's time to be free of the weight of your guilt and shame, talk to Him about it and consider praying something like this:

My God and my Creator,

I have come to believe that You are a God of forgiveness. Your Word and the Cross make it clear that I am forgiven for all the sin I have done, all the sin I am doing, and all the sin I will do in the future. Thank You again for that, Lord. Thanks for making me a forgiven person.

But Father, I've been unable and unwilling to forgive myself for ____ (List them out for Him! All of them!) I now see that it's destructive and wrong not to forgive myself, and I want to be free from the harm that this is bringing to me and those around me. I also see how this dishonors You, saying your sacrifice on the cross wasn't enough, and robs You of my praise and worship.

God, I can't forgive myself for these things on my own. I need You to move in my life, giving me the faith, the desire, and the strength to forgive myself. I ask that You would do that now. By Your strength, I forgive myself and declare myself free from these sins because You have forgiven me.

When my feelings try to drag me back into guilt and self-condemnation, please quickly remind me of who I am as Your child. Continually remind me that I've been completely cleansed and forgiven of these things, no matter how I feel.

Lord, I praise You and I thank You for this new freedom! Lead me now, guide me now and empower me to live as You desire.

Amen.

Seeking Forgiveness from Others

One last area of forgiveness completes the powerful healing process. When you have sinned against someone else, consider the words of Matthew 5:23-24:

Therefore if you are presenting your offering at the altar,
and there remember that your brother has something against you,
leave your offering there before the altar and go;
first be reconciled to your brother...

When you have wronged another, and the other person knows it or has suffered in anyway from your actions, now is the time to ask for forgiveness. *Now*, not later. The pattern in Matthew suggests that even your normal routine of worship and service should be interrupted if you need to seek reconciliation from someone you have offended.

These basic steps will help guide you—but you will want to listen to the specific guidance of God as you approach the person you have hurt.

1. Clearly identify what you did and the impact it had on the other person.
2. Thank God for forgiving you, because ultimately, the sin is against Him.

3. Ask the person you sinned against to forgive you. Be specific. Don't just say, "I'm sorry." Ask, "Will you forgive me for _____?" Those four words, "Will you forgive me?" are perhaps the hardest to say of any words that exist. Freedom always comes with a price. Forgiveness comes with humility. Asking for forgiveness is tremendously awkward, and your flesh will fight to avoid it. But I am telling you that it is worth it. When you pick up the telephone and say those four words, healing from your actions takes place in your heart. If they forgive you, healing takes place in their heart as well.

4. If the person extends forgiveness, you are free from the sin...and so are they (if they follow God's example and take your sin to the cross). If they don't forgive you, you are still free, and the other person will have to carry the weight of your sin and suffer the consequences of unresolved anger.

This process may not release you from the earthly consequences of your actions, however. You may still face serious legal or financial ramifications because of what you did. One of the consequences may be living with a broken relationship. There is no guarantee that the person you have hurt is going to forgive you. The relational implications of your actions could be severing and severe. But no matter what you've done or continue to do, *it's never too late to do the right thing—and seeking forgiveness is always the right thing.*

Embracing the forgiveness of God; forgiving others; forgiving yourself; seeking forgiveness from those you have wronged-these are the privileges, the rights, and the responsibilities of those who walk in the shadow of the cross. Forgiveness is a gift of God, designed by Him, modeled by the Son, and paid for by His blood. May all of us have the wisdom to daily allow the forgiveness of Christ to flow to us and through us.

If possible, so far as it depends on you, be at peace with all men.
ROMANS 12:18

After meeting with Bill, Karen and Richard took a long walk in the park. They had much to talk about as they reflected on how Richard's decision to have a beer while on duty had affected their lives. There was so much they had learned. At a picnic table under a large oak tree, they took out a sheet of paper and began their lists. Karen wrote down how Richard's actions had blocked her desires to begin a family. He wrote down how devastating Karen's judgmental reaction had made him feel. He wrote down how the decision of the chief seemed unfair in light of his perfect record. She wrote down her thoughts toward the officer who had turned him in...and then taken his promotion. When the list of others' offenses against them were complete, they thanked God for the Cross, asked Him to extend His forgiveness through them, renounced their desires to punish, and tore up the lists-letting the small pieces of paper drift away on the wind.

Turning to each other, they then confessed their sins toward each other. Karen apologized for the way she had vented her anger through harsh words and withholding affection. Richard apologized for the way that his actions had hurt her and dashed her hopes to be a stay-at-home mom. She confessed how her spending habits had pulled them into debt. When it was all out, each asked, "Will you forgive me?" and each heard the reply of true reconciliation, "Yes, I forgive you." As Karen said those words, she began to breathe normally for the first time in months.

Finally, Richard asked God to make him willing to forgive himself. And as he did so, he could feel the anger and stress being released from his shoulders.

From the park they drove to a restaurant that was popular with the police force. After buying gift certificates, they wrote anonymous letters to the chief and the new sergeant, thanking them for their service to the community and for the way they had personally impacted their lives. They sealed and sent the letters with sincere prayer for God's blessings to be on these two men.

On the way home, Karen slid her hand into Richard's and he held it tightly. Together they started working out a possible plan for reducing their debt and creating a second source of income that would allow Karen to stay at home. Together they decided that it was probably still best to wait to have children ... but apparently Someone had other plans. That night, their first son slipped unnoticed into their lives.

Therefore if anyone is in Christ, he is a new creature;
the old things passed away; behold, new things have come.
Now all these things are from God, who reconciled us to Himself
through Christ and gave us the ministry of reconciliation, namely,
that God was in Christ reconciling the world to Himself,
not counting their trespasses against them, and He has committed
to us the word of reconciliation.

2 CORINTHIANS 5:17-19

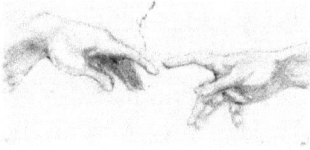

CHAPTER 5

Rest for the Soul;
Power for Life

"Come to Me, all who are weary and heavy-laden,

and I will give you rest... for I am gentle and humble in heart,

and you will find rest for your souls.

MATTHEW 11:28-29

In the first book of the New Testament, Matthew records a beckoning invitation that Christ made to the masses of people in the cities He visited. The call and the invitation have resonated in the hearts of billions of people: the tired, the burned out, and the lost. The call has gone out for thousands of years, on every continent, to tens of thousands of different tribes and nations. "Come to Me," He said, "all who are weary and heavy-laden, and I will give you rest. Take My yoke upon you and learn from Me, for I am gentle and humble in heart, and you will find rest for your souls" (Matthew 11:28-30).

The call comes to us at an important junction. The dark and draining errors of our ways have been identified and dealt with at the Cross.

Forgiveness now frees us from the past, allowing us to look with expectation toward the future. A new and different way of living awaits us, a way that frees us from the burdens of circumstance and stress. He calls us to come, and He promises us *rest* for our souls. He has also promised that, "You will know the truth, and the truth will make you free" (John 8:32).

Three foundations of truth lay at the base of His promises for rest and freedom. If we misunderstand any one of them, we will be launched back into lives of self-effort and stress. If we come to understand them, however, and allow them to soak into our dry and thirsty souls, we will begin to discover a river of cool, satisfying water that continually refreshes and renews us.

Come to Jesus now, and discover the new way He has designed for us to walk. Find comfort in the three areas of truth that will serve as a solid rock of protection against the storms of life. May your soul find rest in all that the Lord is, in all that the Lord has done, and in all that He has made you to be. *This is the true answer to our stressful lives.* The peace that we all so desperately seek in our lives is really found in these three truths.

TRUTH #1: Rest in Who He Is

*What comes to mind when we think about God
is the most important thing about us.*

A. W. TOZER

> **When it comes to the health of our soul, nothing is more important than our beliefs about God.**

When it comes to the health of our soul, nothing is more important than our beliefs about God. I'm not talking about what we say we believe, but what we *really* believe, deep down inside. These beliefs rarely reveal themselves in normal circumstances. It's during the storms of life that our true beliefs are forced to the surface. Will our souls find rest when all hell seems to be breaking loose around us? It all depends on what we really believe about God. Here are just some of the attributes of God that allow us to find rest:

God Loves

Our beliefs about the love of God may be the most important of all the beliefs we have about Him, and they permeate every other belief we hold. The Bible is rich in its proclamation and description of His passionate affection for us. Consider these passages:

- His love for us is as high as the heavens are above the earth (Psalm 103:11).
- His love is sacrificial, even to the point of death (John 3:16; Hebrews 12:2).
- His love is demonstrated at the cross (Romans 5:8).
- His love is inseparable. Nothing can take it away from us (Romans 8:35-39).
- His love is gracious and great (Ephesians 2:4).
- The love of Christ surpasses knowledge (Ephesians 3:19).

The belief in God's love for us is the beginning of finding rest for our souls. While God's love extends to the whole world, He also focuses this love like a laser beam on one specific target: you! It's hard to fathom, I know. But His love is so personal, His affections for you are so intentional, that had you been the only person to walk upon this earth, He still would have come to earth to walk with you, and then sacrificed Himself for your sin, that He might be able to enjoy your company now and into eternity. His love is that intense. His love is that deliberate.

God Is Holy

When the Bible says that God is "holy", it means that God is "sacred" and "set apart" in a way that has no possible earthly comparison. In 1 Samuel 2:2, Hannah proclaimed, "There is no one holy like the LORD, Indeed, there is no one besides You. Nor is there any rock like our God."

- God is absolutely perfect, just, faithful, and righteous (Deuteronomy 32:1-4).
- God has all power and nothing is too hard for Him to do (Jeremiah 32:17; 27).

Our peace should grow in knowing that a loving God is also perfect in all His ways. He makes no mistakes. He overlooks no detail.

God Forgives

Left to our own merit and our own performance, it's easy to see that a holy God would have no choice other than to punish us and separate us from His pure sacredness. Oh, how we should praise Him for the Cross! With His perfect sacrifice, He paid the full penalty of our sin. With justice, righteousness, and without any compromise to His holiness, He has forgiven us and reconciled us to Him.

We can rest in the fact that a loving and holy God has also received us and accepted us!

God Provides

So much of our stress and worry come from our fear of the future. When we face financial challenges, sickness, or threats to our physical and emotional security, our souls can be protected by the belief that God is a perfect provider.

- God owns everything and all resources are at His wise disposal (Psalm 50:10-12).
- God knows what we need (Matthew 6:31-32).
- God is a generous God, even to the unrighteous (Acts 14:16-17).
- God supplies all our needs (Philippians 4:19).

The startling implication of this is not just the promise that God *will* provide what we need, but that He is providing all we need. If we really believe that God is a loving, holy, and forgiving Provider, then we can rest in the fact that all things *are* working out for our good (Romans 8:28), even when we can't see it in outward circumstances, even when we face things that are clearly "bad" or even "evil."

God Is in Control

Psalm 103:19-22 says, "The LORD has made the heavens His throne; from there He rules everything ... Praise the LORD, everything He created, everywhere in His kingdom." Paul echoes this in his first letter to Timothy, "He who is the blessed and only Sovereign, the King of kings and the Lord of lords, who alone possesses immortality and dwells in unapproachable light ... to Him be honor and eternal dominion!" (1 Timothy 6:15-16)

God is not just in control of the circumstances around us; He is also in control of the changes taking place in us. Isaiah 45:5-10 describes us as lumps of clay and God as a potter who is molding us and shaping us. This can be a difficult process as God stretches and tears us, squishes us and spins us. The firm and gentle work of His hands upon our lives is the very best thing for us as we learn to rest in who He is, and who He is making us to be. Romans 8:29 tells us that He is conforming us into to the image of Jesus Himself, with the result that He will be recognized as more important than anyone else.

Do you see the pattern here? *God is in control, and He is doing it in a way that will bring ultimate glory and praise to Himself, the only one to whom praise is due.*

If you heed the call of Jesus to come and find rest, you will find that rest for your soul begins in a heartfelt belief in the truth about who God is. He is loving, holy, and forgiving. He is a perfect provider and He is in control.

TRUTH #2: Rest in What He Has Done

True rest begins with a practical belief in the character of God. After that, though, rest finds fuel in what the Lord has done. These are things that are already completed, things that He has already accomplished in His holy perfection. I need to warn you that as we explore what God has done, you may not see evidence of it in your life yet. The realization of these things will begin to manifest itself after you believe them and begin to allow God to make them practical realities in your outward life. It's all part of His design; it's all part of His perfect plan that has been unfolding since the dawn of time.

Let's take a look at Romans 8:28-30 to gain a broader perspective on what God has done:

> *We know that God causes all things to work together*
> *for good to those who love God, to those who are called*
> *according to His purpose. [That's you!] For those whom He foreknew,*
> *He also predestined to become conformed to the image of His Son,*
> *so that He would be the firstborn among many brethren;*
> *and these whom He predestined [That's you!] He also called,*
> *and these whom He called, He also justified;*
> *and these whom He justified, He also glorified.*

These are all powerful words: "predestined, called, justified, glorified." We could write entire books on each one! The key we want you to see, however, is that He did them. Every good thing that we are is from His effort, not our self-effort! Keep an eye out for this as you read your Bible. You'll see that He Is the one who has already done so many of the things that we normally strive to do on our own.

For example, 1 Corinthians 1:29-31 says "... no man may boast before God. But by His doing you are in Christ Jesus, who became to us wisdom from God, and righteousness and sanctification, and redemption, so that, just as it is written, 'Let him who boasts, boast in the LORD.' "

Do you see the ramifications of this? The Bible says because of what

God did, we are *already* in Christ, and Christ has *already* become our righteousness, our purification, and our salvation. Second Corinthians 1:21-22 says *God* is the one who established us "in Christ," who "anointed" us, "sealed" us and "gave us the Spirit in our hearts as a pledge." Ephesians 1:3-6 says that *God* has "blessed us with every spiritual blessing", that *God* "chose us in Him before the foundation of the world", that *He* freely bestowed on us His grace.

We could go on and on. Each specific blessing that God has given us is tremendously important. But again, the general belief that you need to see is that He is the one who did it all; it's all past tense...and in that truth we can rest.

TRUTH #3: Rest in Who He Has Made You to Be

As amazing as God is and as incredible as the things are that He has done for you, the intimate truths concerning what He has done to you may be the most astounding. Prayerfully ponder the following passages. Even if you are familiar with what they say, search your heart to see if you *really* believe them, even in very small measure:

- Do you not know that you are a temple of God and that the Spirit of God dwells in you? (1 Corinthians 3:16)
- I have been crucified with Christ, and it is no longer I who live, but Christ who lives in me. (Galatians 2:20)
- Because you are sons, God has sent forth the Spirit of His Son into our hearts... (Galatians 4:6)
- But God, being rich in mercy, because of His great love with which He loved us, even when we were dead in our transgressions, made us alive together with Christ. (Ephesians 2:4-5)
- And we know that the Son of God has come, and has given us understanding so that we may know Him who is true; and we are in Him who is true, in His Son Jesus Christ. (1 John 5:20)

> Ceasing from self-effort is only the first step out of bondage. Victory comes when we allow Christ Himself to live His life through us. We vacate, He occupies, and then He begins to live the very life He designed us to live through us.

Do you grasp the implications of passages like these? The Bible says that when you asked Christ into your life, God really came in...really. An exchange of life has taken place. God's Spirit has taken up residence in your spirit.

You no longer live unto yourself. Christ lives in you.

This is not some minor theological detail. This is the core of the most practical realities that a follower of Christ can realize. When—and only when—this truth is recognized and applied can you enter into the perpetual rest and obedience that God has made available. Ceasing from self-effort is only the first step out of bondage. Victory comes when we allow Christ Himself to live His life through us. We vacate, He occupies, and then He begins to live the very life He designed us to live through us.

Resting in the Lord is so very much more than surrender. As we give Him control, our days become very powerful, very active, and our rest is experienced in His activity. That's the key to praying "without ceasing" (1 Thessalonians 5:17). It's simply a moment-by-moment awareness of the constant presence of Christ in our life. It's the key to "walking in the Spirit." *We walk not to get closer to the Spirit of God, but we walk because the Spirit already lives within us.*

You are in Him and He is in you! This truth is miraculous, mysterious, and yet one of the most powerful and practical truths that you can believe. It changes the way you can think about anything and the way you do everything. God has done it all and He continues to do it all...and that opens the door to a completely new way to live.

> ...if anyone is in Christ, he is a new creature;
> the old things passed away; behold, new things have come.
> Now all these things are from God,
> who reconciled us to Himself through Christ...
> 2 CORINTHIANS 5:17-18

New Things Have Come

> What can we attain without effort? How can we ever
> get anywhere if we do not move? But Christianity is a strange business!
> If at the outset we try to do anything, we get nothing;
> if we seek to attain something, we miss everything.
> For Christianity begins not with a big DO but a big DONE.
> WATCHMAN NEE, *SIT WALK STAND*

Let's get a few things straight before we continue. First, when we were born again, God didn't "adjust" us, "tweak" us, or give us a "tune up." *He killed us and started over again.* Our flesh may still be living by old habits, but in our spirits (the very core of our beings) we are brand new.

Second, when we now approach the Christian life, we are not to just "adjust", "tweak", or "tune up" our old ways of doing things. When Christ calls us to rest in Him, He is calling us to an entirely new way of living. He hasn't renovated or cleaned up our old life. He has destroyed it. Resting in the Lord is trusting in who He is, what He has done, and who He has made us to be. The supernatural peace and absence of stress in our lives that results is an attribute of a new life. Resting is an extension of who we already are, by God; it's not trying to be something we are not. It starts with stopping, and even the things that we do are done totally differently.

Resting in the Lord Leads to Peace

The opposite of stress and anxiety is peace. When you begin resting in the Lord and abiding in Christ, you will experience a supernatural peace that Scripture tells you will protect your heart and mind. "And the peace of God, which surpasses all comprehension, will guard your hearts and your minds in Christ Jesus" (Philippians 4:7). What is going on in your spirit and your soul does affect your body either for the good or for the bad. When you are resting in the Lord, His supernatural peace brings a calmness that truly affects your health. The level of your stress hormones decrease, your blood pressure decreases, your pulse rate and respiratory rate slow down, and your immune system actually strengthens. It is just the opposite result of what stress does to your body. A natural healing occurs when we are supernaturally resting in Christ!

> **When you are resting in the Lord, His supernatural peace brings a calmness that truly affects your health.**

If only I could count the number of sincere Christians that have come into my examining room or Bill's counseling center still trying to live the old way. Their new lives in Christ held out so much promise to them, but they have found only disillusionment, illness, and despair. No, God calls us to something new, something we were designed for, and He gives us a picture of it in John 15:4-5:

> *Abide in Me, and I in you. As the branch cannot bear fruit*
> *of itself unless it abides in the vine, so neither can you unless*

you abide in Me. I am the vine and you are the branches;
he who abides in Me and I in Him, he bears much fruit,
for apart from Me you can do nothing.

That is the secret to living a successful Christian life. Success is not found in what you have done, nor is it found in who you have made yourself out to be. Success, victory, rest, and peace are found in an "abiding" relationship with Jesus. To abide means "to live, dwell, and exist in something." Just as a grape branch withers, shrivels, and dies when it is severed from the vine, so our lives deteriorate and die when we try to live independently from Jesus. But in an abiding relationship with the Lord we find peace, power, purpose, passion, and reason to praise.

Some might object to this idea, thinking that "rest" is the absence of work, and that we are to be about the Lord's work. But resting in the Lord is infinitely more than just ceasing our self-effort. Resting in the Lord consumes us with God, unleashes His vision and power within us, and launches us into a new life of focus and victory where we carry only the burdens that He designed us to carry. When it comes to doing His work, those who rest in Him are the most productive of all, because He is the one who works through them!

Resting in the Lord consumes us with God, unleashes His vision and power within us, and launches us into a new life of focus and victory where we carry only the burdens that He designed us to carry.

As Jesus calls us to find rest for our souls in Matthew 11:29-30, He uses an interesting illustration. He says, "Take My yoke upon you.... For My yoke is easy and My burden is light." A yoke is a wooden beam that is strapped across the shoulders of an animal, helping it to pull or carry heavy loads. The first indication that we are carrying our own yoke is that it is heavy and stressful. That's the sign that we are living by self-effort, perhaps carrying a concern that isn't ours.

Before you can take on the restful yoke of Christ that is easy and light, we first have to take off the old yoke. This is the first and all-important beginning that will be followed by the need to renew the mind to truth, applying biblical principles and following clear commands of Scripture. But in every situation we face, we must begin from a position of rest, rather than self-effort. Scripture is very clear that believers build up strongholds one block at a time. When we begin to tear down these strongholds in our life, they must also be torn down one block at a time as we begin renewing our mind and abiding in Christ.How do you do that? Let's look at three examples; however, remember that this is just the beginning of the process.

Jim has been struggling with Internet pornography. He has been trying and failing, trying and failing, in his attempts to stop. He constantly feels separated from God and filthy inside. He has recently realized that he has been going at it all wrong. Finally, he gives up and offers this prayer:

"God, I've been trying to fight this in my own strength and I've failed. Thank You that You have already forgiven me of this sin and paid for it, in full, at the Cross. Lord, I give up the battle and put my trust in You and Your Word. The Bible says that You have already made me clean. I am clean! I am Your son! You live in me right at this very moment! I ask You to focus my mind and thoughts on who You are. Free me from my own attempts to win this fight on my own. I rest in You. You are my God! I worship You and praise You!"

Linda is completely exhausted. She's been trying as hard as she can to be a good mom. She's been trying to be a good wife. She volunteers at school and church. Deep down inside she feels like she still isn't doing enough. She is afraid that people are already disappointed in her, and she wonders if God still accepts her as she flounders in her service to Him. One day her pastor asks her to teach a Sunday school class. With nothing left to give she wants to say "no", but instead she feels compelled to say "yes." In her exhaustion, she calls out to God:

"Oh, my Lord, I've done it again! I've allowed demands to draw me away from You and Your truth. I've given in to the pressures that tell me I must "do, do, do" to be accepted by others and You. In the process I've shut You out and tried to do it all on my own. I'm sorry! Thanks for forgiving me. You have already made me completely acceptable. In You I am loved, forgiven, directed, and embraced by You, my perfect Father. Thank You that I can abide in You right now. I don't want to be driven by the demands and expectations of those around me. Guide me and lead me in my choices. Show me what things You want to do together, as I rest in Your arms again."

William has just gotten fired from his job. The timing is not good. There are bills to pay and unexpected expenses at home. As he sits at home, wondering what to do, he can feel the fear and anxiety welling up inside his soul.

As he begins to feel the weight of his situation, He lifts his head and hands toward heaven and begins to talk to his Father.

> "Oh, God, this is not what I had planned, and I don't know what to do; I don't know what to think. I'm afraid, Lord. Jesus, I know that You are here, and I know that Your Spirit is inside me. More than that, I know that I am not even my own. My life is Your life; Your life is my life. I depend fully on You to live out this situation as You see fit. I release it all into your hands and rest in the truth that You are my perfect provider. I trust not only in the fact that you will provide for me in the future, but that You are providing for me right now by giving me this situation to mold me into Your image. By Your power, I even rejoice in what has happened! You are a holy God, and God who is in control!"

The New Battle

The writer of the book of Hebrews left us with a very interesting warning and a new challenge. In this unusual passage, he lays out a new battle plan for the Christian life:

> Therefore, let us fear if, while a promise remains of entering His rest, any one of you may seem to have come short of it. For indeed we have had good news preached to us... we who have believed enter that rest.... Therefore, since it remains for some to enter it, and those who formerly had good news preached to them failed to enter because of disobedience ... For the one who has entered His rest has himself also rested from his own works.... Therefore let us be diligent to enter that rest, so that no one will fall, through following the same example of disobedience.
>
> HEBREWS 4:1-6, 10-11

This passage takes resting in the Lord from being a "nice option" to being a clear command...with fearful implications for those who disobey and continue in the self-effort of their own works. It calls us to "be diligent" to enter rest so that we don't fall into disobedience. Certainly we have a clear choice to make. We can actively choose to enter God's rest at any time; or we can choose to stress, worry, and flounder in self-effort. In fact, if we really believe the good news that was preached to us about who God is, what He has done, and who He has already made us to be, this passage says we *will* enter that rest.

But let there be no mistake. Entering the rest of the Lord is a battle. Satan will attempt to distract you; he might try to fill your thoughts with doubt about God's character, what He has done, and what He will do. The world will continually attempt to pull you away from rest and persuade you to go back to self-effort in order to get what it says you need to be happy and fulfilled.

Your battle plan is to fight with faith and truth, standing firm on what the Word says is true. As in the examples above, you can always come back to rest in the midst of difficult times. Better yet, however, would be an ongoing strategy that keeps you firmly grounded in a state of rest before the attacks come.

How do you do that? Ask God to do something new! Ask Him to stir up a desire for a regular time of focused rest—a time when the two of you get away from the distractions of the world and talk and relax in each other's presence. A time when you can contemplate what is true, what is right, and what is good. A time when you can focus on Him in uninterrupted praise, worship of who He is, what He has done, and what He has made you to be. In these times, the truth is solidified in your heart, giving you strength that can permeate the most demanding of days.

The Ramifications of Rest
Peace

Philippians 4:4-7 calls us to "rejoice in the Lord always," bringing Him our thanksgiving and our requests. When we do, He promises that our anxieties will be replaced by "the peace of God, which surpasses all comprehension, will guard your hearts and minds in Christ Jesus." This is the peace everyone is seeking, but few find. Peace is there for the believer who learns to trust God and place their faith in Him. When you surrender your will to God and His indwelling Holy Spirit, you will find it. His promise is the fact that He will supernaturally protect and guard your body (physical heart) and soul (mind).

Power

God designed us to find strength and ability in our rest and complete dependence in Him. He knows that even as we rest in Him, we will continue to face great opposition, trials, and pain in the world.

Second Corinthians 4:7-9 reassures us about the sufficiency of God in the face of difficulty, affirming that "the surpassing greatness of the power will be of God and not from ourselves; we are afflicted in every way, but not crushed; perplexed, but not despairing; persecuted but not forsaken; struck down but not destroyed...." Even the apostle Paul—who saw great victory and great difficulty in his ministry—confessed that it was God who was at work. "But by the grace of God I am what I am, and His grace toward me did not prove vain; but I labored even more than all of them, yet not I, but the grace of God with me" (1 Corinthians 15:10).

Paul's understanding of the power of God for those who rest in Him led him to offer this prayer for the people of Ephesus: "For this reason I bow my knees before the Father, from whom every family in heaven and on earth derives its name, that He would grant you, according to the riches of His glory, to be strengthened with power through His Spirit in the inner man, so that Christ may dwell in your hearts through faith; and that you, being rooted and grounded in love, may be able to comprehend with all the saints what is the breadth and length and height and depth, and to know the love of Christ which surpasses knowledge, that you may be filled up to all the fullness of God (Ephesians 3:14-19).

Purpose

Those who truly rest in the Lord find no reason to be lazy or complacent. Quite to the contrary, rest focuses our hearts on the things of God. It's like the runner that focuses on the finish line or the golfer that focuses on the flag and the cup. When we rest in who He is and what He has done, we are drawn toward the things that are on His heart. Rest leads us into an intimacy with Him where His plans overflow into our hopes and dreams.

The one who rests in the Lord comes to understand that "we are His workmanship, created in Christ Jesus for good works, which God prepared beforehand so that we would walk in them" (Ephesians 2:10). The one who rests in the Lord also finds freedom from the worries of the world. As you recognize God as the perfect provider, anxieties about what to eat, what to drink, and what to wear are absorbed into the belief that "your heavenly Father knows that you need all these things, but seek first His kingdom and His righteousness, and all these things will be added to you" (Matthew 6:32-33).

Passion

Resting in the Lord also increases our passion for the things of God. The natural resting response puts our minds at ease and into a state where we are more receptive to the Word and the Spirit. Focusing on Him allows us to filter out other voices and hear more clearly what He is saying moment by moment.

Significantly, when we come to really rest in His love for us, we will naturally come to love others. In fact, the Scriptures tell us that we can *only* love others because He first loved us (1 John 4:19). As we begin to return His love, the Word promises "you will keep My commandments" (John 14:15). That love can come only from resting in who He is and what He has done. The moment we try to love Him on our own, the purity of His grace is "disgraced," and we fall back into the trap of self-effort.

Praise

Finally, a life lived in rest brings ultimate praise to God, rather than self. Ephesians 1:5-6 says that God has adopted us "through Jesus Christ to Himself, according to the kind intention of His will, to the praise of the glory of His grace...." Ephesians 1:12 confirms that we have obtained God's inheritance "to the end that we who were the first to hope in Christ should be to the praise of His glory."

First Corinthians 1:30-31 makes it extra clear, giving full credit to God for the things He has done. "But by His doing you are in Christ Jesus... that, just as it is written, 'Let him who boasts, boast in the LORD."

Revelation four paints an extreme, graphic picture of the praise that will erupt in heaven on the day when people from every tribe, every tongue, and every nation bow before the Lord. On that day heavenly creatures will shout out day and night proclaiming, "Holy, Holy, Holy is the LORD GOD, the Almighty!" (Revelation 4:8). In that moment, in a symbolic gesture of their understanding of God's work through their rest, twenty-four elders (who have just received crowns of reward for their faithful service) will cast those crowns before the throne of the Lord saying, "Worthy are You, our Lord and our God, to receive glory and honor and power; for You created all things, and because of Your will they existed, and were created" (Revelation 4:10-11). We will all be there on that day. But there is no reason to wait until then! Right here, right now, you can rest in the Lord. You can rest in who He is, in what He has done, and in what He has made you to be.

Rest in the Lord and the things of the earth will grow strangely dim.

Bask in His presence as His child and know His peace and His healing strength. Rest in the Lord and His power, purpose, and passion will be released into your weary and heavy laden soul.

For this reason also, since the day we heard of it,
we have not ceased to pray for you and to ask that you
may be filled with the knowledge of His will in all spiritual wisdom
and understanding, so that you will walk in a manner worthy
of the Lord, to please Him in all respects, bearing fruit in
every good work and increasing in the knowledge of God;
strengthened with all power, according to His glorious might,
for the attaining of all steadfastness and patience;
joyously giving thanks to the Father, who has qualified us
to share in the inheritance of the saints in Light.
COLOSSIANS 1:9-12

For an expanded discussion on these all important topics, read Rest Assured, by Bill Ewing, Real Life Press, 2003.

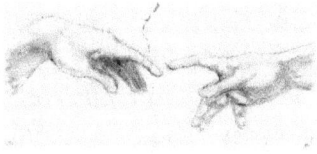

CHAPTER 6

Rest at War— the Battle for the Mind

Stand firm against the schemes of the devil.

For our struggle is not against flesh and blood ...

EPHESIANS 6:11-12

George could feel his heart pounding as the lush green foliage of a small Pacific island grew steadily in the windshield of his plane. *From a distance, the island looked like a small paradise floating in the midst of the crystal clear skies and the deep blues of the ocean. But George and his crew knew that they were headed for no vacation. To a casual observer, Chichi Jima might have seemed like an insignificant destination, but this was September 1944 and this small dot on the map held a crucial target as the battles of World War II reached a climax.*

Chichi Jima was only about two-and-a-half miles wide and five- miles long, but its peaks were crowded with radio towers and antennas. On the ridges and in the valleys 25,000 soldiers manned machine guns and anti- aircraft batteries to protect the stations on the peaks that housed the enemies' transmitters and receivers.

The stations had been intercepting and interfering with U.S. military communications and they were a strategic information link between Tokyo and other Japanese-held islands. Both sides knew that whoever controlled the messages from the stations would control the region. Destruction of the stations would be a turning point in the largest war ever fought on earth.

As George forced his plane into a shallow dive, menacing clouds of black smoke began erupting all around. He steadied his grip on the control stick but all at once the plane was jolted forward and began to shake violently. As smoke poured from his engines and flames began lapping at the thin skins of his fuel tanks, he managed to keep his sites on the radio stations and released 2,000 pounds of bombs on target. Now he was piloting a falling inferno, still under control, but dropping out of the sky at 190 miles per hour with two crew members in back. In order to give them as much time as possible to parachute to safety, George didn't bail out until the last possible moment. Badly bruised and nearly captured, the twenty year old was eventually rescued from the sea by a submarine.

He was just one of thousands of Americans who fought the battle for the communications center on Chichi Jima. His two crew members were never heard from again. Forty-five years later, George became the forty-first president of the United States.

Today, a massive battle is still being fought over the control of information and truth. The Enemy maintains a position of strength that has gone largely unchallenged. His message of destruction has been transmitted without interference. His communications have been relayed, fortified and hidden by those who knowingly and unknowingly protect and support him. *But this time, the battlefield is not a small Pacific island. Today, the battlefield is your mind.* Just as Chichi Jima held the key to victory in the World War II, winning the battle for your mind is key to victory in life.

Is that a dramatic exaggeration? No, not at all. Not when you understand the crucial, central role of the mind. Your mind is the communications hub for a huge amount of information that is received from the brain, body, and spirit. It controls the will and all decisions regarding life, faith, attitude, and choice. These choices determine the course of our existence. The mind can override emotions. It's the gateway to our relationship with God. It's where our commitment to the King and the kingdom is made and lived out. It's no wonder that the human mind is where the battle rages the strongest, where Satan so desperately seeks to maintain his occupation and control. If he can maintain deception or neutralize your mind, the battle is his.

While we naturally see our battles as being against people, politics, or other religions, the Bible shows us differently. By design, we have been made spirit, soul, and body. Separate and yet inseparable, a scriptural understanding of who we are is important as we seek to identify our enemies...and our ultimate Enemy is not one that we can see:

> For though we walk in the flesh, we do not war according to the flesh,
> for the weapons of our warfare are not of the flesh,
> but divinely powerful for the destruction of fortresses.
> We are destroying speculations and every lofty
> thing raised up against the knowledge of God, and we are
> taking every thought captive to the obedience of Christ.
> 2 CORINTHIANS 10:3-5

Satan is a liar and "the father of lies" (John 8:44) and is dedicated to the destruction of our souls through controlling our speculations, knowledge, and thoughts. He is evil, but he is not a fool. He knows that if he can lead our minds astray, everything else is his—and the incredible beauty of what God has done will be shrouded again in our self-effort and self-righteousness. The apostle Paul was deeply concerned about this when he wrote to the Corinthians:

> ...for I betrothed you to one husband, so that to Christ
> I might present you as a pure virgin. But I am afraid that,
> as the serpent deceived Eve by his craftiness, that your minds
> will be led astray from the simplicity and purity of devotion to Christ.
> 2 CORINTHIANS 11:2-3

Please grasp the significance of this. Paul has shared the truth of the Gospel with them and has walked them down the aisle toward a beautiful and innocent relationship with Christ. But he's afraid; afraid that the Evil One will pollute, distort, and deceive them, pulling them away from a simple, resting dedication to Jesus. What is the core of Paul's concern? "...that your minds will be led astray".

True transformation comes from taking back Enemy ground in our mind and establishing a fortress of God's truth in our hearts. When we renew the mind, we confront lies and then replace them with truth.

We don't have to look far to see that Satan has succeeded with this strategy in the past. In fact, at one point in history it got so bad that, "the LORD saw that the wickedness of man was great on the earth, and that every intent of the thoughts of his heart was only evil continually" (Genesis 6:5). It was so bad that God put His few remaining followers on a boat, flooded the earth, and started over.

Just as an enemy controlled the flow of information from Chichi Jima more than sixty years ago, today Satan's aim is to control the human mind. Will you be brave enough to attack the fortresses of evil, "destroying speculations and every lofty thing raised up against the knowledge of God, taking every thought captive?"

An Offensive Transformation.

Romans 12:2 calls us into battle with this challenge:

Do not be conformed to this world, but be transformed
by the renewing of your mind, so that you may prove
what the will of God is, that which is good and acceptable and perfect.

True transformation comes from taking back Enemy ground in our mind and establishing a fortress of God's truth in our hearts. When we renew the mind, we confront lies and then replace them with truth. Established in truth, our minds will begin to make decisions that align with God's design, maximizing our lives for the things that matter the most now and in eternity. Ephesians 4:17-18; 20-24 uses these words to alert us to the battle for our minds:

...walk no longer just as the Gentiles also walk, in the futility of their mind,
being darkened in their understanding, excluded from the life of God because
of the ignorance that is in them, because of the hardness of their heart;...
But you did not learn Christ in this way, if indeed you have heard Him and
have been taught in Him, just as truth is in Jesus, that, in reference to your
former manner of life, you lay aside the old self, which is being corrupted in
accordance with the lusts of deceit, and that you be renewed in the spirit of
your mind, and put on the new self, which in the likeness of God has been
created in righteousness and holiness of the truth.

Those are our marching orders, our call to do battle. God has designed us for a passionate and resting relationship with Him—but a barrage of lies and half-truths continually bombard us, driving us back into self-effort, stress, and independence from Jesus. We are to rebel against these messages, claim the truth about who God is, what He has done, and who He has made us to be. Thankfully, the Scriptures give us clear instructions of how this is to be done:

> Be anxious for nothing, but in everything by prayer
> and supplication with thanksgiving let your requests be
> made known to God. And the peace of God, which surpasses all
> comprehension, will guard your hearts and your minds in Christ Jesus.
> Finally, brethren, whatever is honorable, whatever is right,
> whatever is pure, whatever is lovely, whatever is of good repute,
> if there is any excellence and if anything worthy of praise,
> dwell on these things. The things you have learned
> and received and heard and seen in me,
> practice these things, and the God of peace will be with you.
>
> PHILIPPIANS 4:6-9

Let's dissect this passage and look at what he's telling us. First, we are to, "be anxious for nothing…" *When anxiety, stress, and fear rear their heads, it's an indicator that our minds are getting the wrong message from somewhere.* Our thoughts are trying to tell us something contrary to truth about God and who we are as His children"…but in everything by prayer and supplication with thanksgiving let your requests be made known to God." ("Supplication" is simply asking God to intervene in some way.) Take those thoughts captive and replace them with thankful praise about God. Thank Him that He is in control of the specific circumstance causing anxiety; thank Him that in His loving-kindness He will use this very occurrence to make your life better than it was before. Then let Him know your requests!

When you leave your concerns with Him, then He does something miraculous. "And the peace of God, which surpasses all comprehension, will guard your hearts and your minds in Christ Jesus." Renewing your thoughts and

> **When you leave your concerns with Him, then He does something miraculous. "And the peace of God, which surpasses all comprehension, will guard your hearts and your minds in Christ Jesus."**

praying about your desires is actually a defense against the onslaught of evil. God's peace will then begin to protect your heart and mind as well as your health.

We are to take an active roll in this process by intentionally focusing our minds on "whatever is honorable, whatever is right, whatever is pure, whatever is lovely, whatever is of good repute, if there is any excellence and if anything worthy of praise, dwell on these things." It's not enough to just get rid of the junk. God wants to replace it with thoughts that are worthy of being pondered in the amazing minds He has given us.

The thoughts that we choose need to meet *all* the criteria listed in this Scripture. It's not always profitable to dwell on things that are only true. (For example, true memories from our past might also be impure or destructive.) We are to focus on the things that are "honorable" and "pure," "lovely", and "worthy of praise".

Finally, we hear this challenge: "The things you have learned and received and heard and seen in Me, practice these things." With our minds now set on what is good and true, we are to activate our wills through choosing a course of action that reflects what the mind says is true. It really is "practice." Setting the mind is an ongoing, moment-by-moment process. We will never do it perfectly, but we are moving in the right direction, empowered by Him, seeking to think as we were designed to think. What's the end result? "The God of peace will be with you."

In short, when you feel yourself being led astray by evil thoughts:
- Recognize the thought as a lie.
- Replace it with prayer and truth, according to Scripture.
- Rejoice in God and your rest in Him.
- Respond with actions that reflect truth.

Setting the Mind

For those who are according to the flesh
set their minds on the things of the flesh, but those
who are according to the Spirit, the things of the Spirit.
ROMANS 8:5

The concept of "setting the mind" is one of the most important in our attack against the strongholds of evil. "Setting the mind" gives us an image of mental steadfastness, stability, and permanence. When our minds are set, they are grounded like the roots of a tall and seasoned oak tree, like an anchor set in concrete.

There is no need to wait around for lies to bombard us before we try to defend ourselves. When we "set our mind" we are taking an offensive position. We take the initiative to saturate our thoughts with the things of the Spirit. In the process, we uproot the strongholds of lies. Because of its incredibly strategic importance, the question must be continually asked, "Where is my mind set right now?"

> **The mind will be set. It's only a question of where it will be set.**

The mind will be set. It's only a question of where it will be set. By default our minds will naturally focus on the things of the flesh, the things we can see, and the things we think we can control. (This usually feels like the natural way to think.)

The flesh draws us into questions such as, "What can others do for me? What can I do in my strength on my own?" The flesh always lures us back into self-effort, manipulating others, and a fearful attempt to manage our circumstances. A sure sign of fleshly thinking is the arguments that we have with others in our minds. You know what we are talking about! We come up with all these things we should have said to really "zing" someone in a past argument, or we start defending ourselves and justifying ourselves about arguments that haven't even taken place yet! If they say that, then we will say this. The whole debate takes place in our imagination (or is played out to a third party) and pretty soon we are as riled up as we would be if it had actually taken place.

Where does it get us? A mind set on the things of the flesh leads us into stress, fear, and tense or broken relationships. Physically the stress of focusing on the flesh sets off the stress reaction, which causes oxidative stress, depletes our immune system, and weakens our health. We've seen how this leads to discouragement, depression, and chronic degenerative disease. This is not a minor "side note" to our existence! Where we set our mind is a matter of life and death for our bodies and our souls:

> *For the mind set on the flesh is death, but the mind set*
> *on the Spirit is life and peace, because the mind set on the flesh*
> *is hostile toward God; for it does not subject itself*
> *to the law of God, for it is not even able to do so,*
> *and those who are in the flesh cannot please God.*
> ROMANS 8:6-8

Through practice, we can actually retrain our minds to automatically think about things of the Spirit. It takes discipline and conscious thought for a while and maybe a good long while. In time, as we take the lead in setting our minds, we can initiate positive change in the right direction. By ongoing choice we have the opportunity to choose to set our minds on the things of the Spirit. When we set our minds on the Spirit, God raises us above the circumstances around us and actually leads us into victory over the things of the flesh. While the flesh will continually try to lure us back into focus on the material, we can choose to let spiritual truth be our standard of reality.

So then, brethren, we are under obligation, not to the flesh...
for if you are living according the flesh,
you must die; but if by the Spirit you are putting to death
the deeds of the body, you will live.
ROMANS 8:12-13

The wonderful thing is that setting our minds on the things of the Spirit is a choice that we can make. Unlike circumstances and people, which are out of our control, setting our minds on the things of the Spirit is something that the Holy Spirit will do in us when we give up and ask Him to do it through us. Sure, *it takes practice and it's something that we need to learn,* but it is clearly within our reach. Paul admitted, "I have learned to be content in whatever circumstances I am.... I have learned the secret of being filled and going hungry, both of having abundance and suffering need. I can do all things through Him who strengthens me" (Philippians 4:11-13).

The Things Above

Colossians 3:1-2 gives us even clearer direction for where to set our minds, "...keep seeking the things above, where Christ is, seated at the right hand of God. Set your mind on the things above, not on the things that are on earth." In what direction are we to set our minds? We are to set them on the truthful things above. What are the things that are above? God, heaven, and you!

God

The Bible is filled with some amazing images of God. As astounding as they are, all of these descriptions fall short of a full image of God. Yet He has revealed Himself in intentional ways for important purposes. Psalm 18, for example, is a song of praise written by David during a time of incredible stress. David was wrapped up "in the cords of death" (v. 4). He said that a bombarding flood "of ungodliness terrified me" (v. 4). Did he fall into despair? No. David knew God, had experienced God as a child and as an adult, and during this time of difficulty raised his eyes to heaven and began to focus on the things above, exposing a daunting image of God:

> In my distress, I called upon the LORD,
> and cried to my God for help.... Then the earth shook
> and quaked; and the foundations of the mountains
> were trembling and were shaken, because He was angry.
> Smoke went up out of His nostrils, and fire from
> His mouth devoured; coals were kindled by it.... The LORD also
> thundered in the heavens, and the Most High uttered His voice,...
> He sent out His arrows, and scattered them, and lightening
> flashes in abundance...He sent from on high, He took me; He drew
> me out of many waters. He delivered me from my strong enemy ...
> PSALM 18:6-8, 13-14, 16-17

When trials come, set your mind on the fact that God is on your side and working in you. He is the very one who is facing your circumstance through you.

That's the kind of God we serve! That's the God who loves us! That's the God whose Spirit lives in you! When trials come, set your mind on the fact that God is on your side and working in you. He is the very one who is facing your circumstance through you.

When David set his mind on God, great strains of praise erupted in his heart. "The Lord lives, and blessed be my rock; and exalted be the God of my salvation..." (Psalm 18:46). It can be the same for you. Make a habit of setting your mind on God. Then, when your flesh is running into anxiousness, you can choose to set your mind on what is above, not on the earth—and the Spirit will replace your worry with worship and wonder. God is near you, with you, and in you. Set your mind on that fact and then let the storms do their worst.

Heaven

As we obey the call to set our minds on the things above, where Christ is, sometimes the image of heaven itself can become a focus of wonder and praise, freeing us from the discouragement of everyday life on earth. Certainly, the earth is passing away and we are destined for much, much better things (Isaiah 51:6). But getting a picture of heaven is not easy! From time to time in history, God opened the eyes of a few men so that they could catch a glimpse of this supernatural place. But when He did, the seers had great difficulty reducing it to human words. Ezekiel is a great example of someone who saw heaven and struggled to communicate its wonders in earthly terms:

> ...while I was by the river Chebar among the exiles,
> the heavens were opened and I saw visions of God...
> As I looked, behold, a storm wind was coming from the north,
> a great cloud with fire flashing forth continually and a
> bright light around it, and in the midst something like glowing metal
> in the midst of the fire. Within it there were figures resembling
> four living beings...In the midst of the living beings there was
> something that looked like burning coals of fire,
> like torches darting back and forth among the living beings...
> the beings ran to and fro like bolts of lightning...
> EZEKIEL 1:1, 4-5, 13-14

In these passages, God has given Ezekiel a powerful, penetrating image of the things of heaven, yet in many cases he can say only that there was an object "something *like* glowing metal," that the figures "*resembled* four living beings," that there was "something that looked *like* burning coals."

Others who were given visions of heaven struggled with the same problem. Heaven is so far beyond earthly comprehension that it has no worldly comparison. But perhaps that's the point! For all of the world's beauty and wonder, don't we long for something beyond this fleshly existence? Something that is above and beyond the daily struggle and decay around us? The vibrant and vivid visions of heaven that God has revealed fuel our hopes with the expectation that there is more going on than meets the eye, that there is someplace else where the battles have been fully won and where peace and power reign in righteousness. We must always remember that heaven is now our true home—not this earthly existence.

Bill has shared with me that when he is faced with difficult thoughts and trials, he directs his attention toward the things above:

Sometimes I picture myself right there, in heaven, as it is described in Ezekiel and Revelation. I bring my thoughts and issues to God, picturing Him taking the concerns from me as I focus on Him in this incredible place. I know my mind can't be set on two things at once. I know I can't carry my own burdens and do His work at the same time. When I leave my concerns at His feet and turn my eyes upon Him, He moves my mind off my issues and me. When He does, I'm moved to love Him, worship Him, and I allow Him to again love others through me.

As we ponder the visions of heaven revealed to us in God's Word, His peace is brought to our weary hearts as well. When we set our mind on heaven above, the things of earth (even the worst things of earth) begin to pale in comparison to the glory that now exists and awaits us.

You!

When we think of setting the mind on "things" above, certainly God and heaven would seem like logical "things". But the Scriptures don't leave it there. We also have descriptions of multitudes of angels and beings that worship the King of kings. We see the dimensions of a great heavenly world that we will, soon enough, inhabit personally. Repeatedly, however, the Bible speaks of an unlikely thing that now exists above, and that is you. Let's consider the fuller context of Colossians 3:1-3:

> **While you may be tempted to discount these words because they seem impossible and outlandish, there is no denying that the Word says that you are a current occupant of "the things above, where Christ is."**

> *Therefore if you have been raised up with Christ,*
> *keep seeking the things above, where Christ is,*
> *seated at the right hand of God. Set your mind on the things above,*
> *not on the things that are on earth. For you have died,*
> *and your life is hidden with Christ in God.*

While you may be tempted to discount these words because they seem impossible and outlandish, there is no denying that the Word says that *you are a current occupant of "the things above, where Christ is."* Note that this condition is not universal to all humans, but "if you have been raised up with Christ...you have died, and your life is hidden with Christ in God." Clearly, you are standing on the edge of something both powerful and mysterious—something that, like heaven and God, transcends your earthly ability to draw a comparison or a parallel—and yet on a spiritual level, you are told to set your mind on these things! You have been crucified with Christ and He now lives in you. He is one of the things above, and because of your relationship with Him, you too are now a citizen of the heavenly places.

The apostle Paul prayed that somehow we might be able to grasp the truth of this mystery:

I pray that the eyes of your heart may be enlightened,
so that you will know what is the hope of His calling,
what are the riches of the glory of His inheritance
in the saints, and what is the surpassing greatness of His power toward us
who believe. These are in accordance
with the working of the strength of His might which
He brought about in Christ, when He raised Him
from the dead and seated Him at His right hand
in the heavenly places...
EPHESIANS 1:18-20.

It's not so difficult to understand that the Bible says Christ was raised from the dead and is now seated in heaven; that's part of the Christian under-standing of Easter. One chapter later, however, we see that God has done the same thing to us!

But God, being rich in mercy, because of His great love
with which He loved us, even when we were dead
in our transgressions, made us alive together with Christ
(by grace you have been saved), and raised us up with Him,
and seated us with Him in the heavenly places in Christ Jesus.
EPHESIANS 2:4-6

God did it to Christ, and now that we are in Christ, He has done it to us as well. Notice that this is all in the past tense! It's not something that *will* happen; it is something that has *already* happened. A mystery? Certainly! A reality? God says it is so. And while the brain may not be able to fathom it, God has designed our souls with the capacity to experience it.

The Power of a Soul at Rest and a Mind that Is Set.

When your soul is "resting in the Lord," God ignites peace, power, purpose, passion, and praise in your heart. "Setting the mind" is really rest at war. A mind set on the things above tears down earthly strongholds, attacks the lies of Satan, and diffuses the strength of our flesh. As a child of the King and a citizen of heaven, when you put the truth into action and set your mind on the Spirit, the repercussions are supernatural. Anxiety and stress no longer control your life nor destroy your health. The true believer in Christ is now capable of experiencing the peace that surpasses all human understanding.

> As a child of the King and a citizen of heaven, when you put the truth into action and set your mind on the Spirit, the repercussions are supernatural.

Freedom!

Jesus said that, "If you continue in My word, then you are truly disciples of Mine; and you will know the truth, and the truth will make you free" (John 8:31-32). Christ has taught us truth. If we choose to live by this truth, applying it as the truth that it is, then a new and radical freedom emerges out of the bondage and burdens we have known.

As our lives become aligned with His design, we find a release from coveting, envy, bitterness, and the desires that cloud our thinking and rob our joy. In *Rose from Brier,* Amy Carmichael described the freedom from circumstances this way.

> *I think this must be important to the clearness of our spiritual atmosphere, for if we let the fugitive wisp of a cloud, which we call a wish (a wish that things were different) float across our sky, then swiftly the whole sweet blue is overcast. But if we refuse that wisp of cloud and look up and meet the love of the Lord that shines down on us, and say to Him about that particular detail of trial, "Dear Lord, yes" then in one bright moment our sky is blue again.*

Setting the mind also gives us the freedom to silence the demanding voices that continually bombard us with expectations. Let's face it: The world is full of people telling us what to do. For many of us, these messages can even echo from the graves of those who have died. Pastors, spouses, advertisers, and parents all try to mold

> Christ has taught us truth. If we choose to live by this truth, applying it as the truth that it is, then a new and radical freedom emerges out of the bondage and burdens we have known.

us according to their desires. Trying to please them only launches us into fear and self-effort.

But the mind set on God knows a peace that gives freedom to the soul. The person who is resting in the Lord is able to cut through the noise and find a place of inner quietness with God where the Word and the Spirit can speak gently and clearly, leading us into specific acts of obedience done in His power. That's ultimate freedom.

Genuine Love

When our hearts are truly resting in the Lord, with our minds set on the things above, it's almost as if we begin to live on a different plane of existence. It's as if our souls are lifted out of all the junk and the pain, and we begin to soak in the most precious of all experiences: Love. *Real* Love. Not the kind of fickle love that dominates the world and all earthly relationships, but the real stuff. The pure, unadulterated, unconditional *agape* love of God. Because His love has no earthly equal, we are again faced with a mighty mystery:

> *We must try to speak of His love. All Christians have tried,*
> *but none have done it very well. I can no more do justice*
> *to that awesome and wonder-filled theme than a child*
> *can grasp a star. Still...as I stretch my heart toward the high,*
> *shining love of God, someone who has not before known*
> *about it may be encouraged to look up and have hope.*
>
> A. W. TOZER, THE KNOWLEDGE OF THE HOLY

Love is like a commodity. We never really own it, but we can trade it. It is never ours to keep, but when we give it away it comes back to us in greater measure. Love is part of God's supernatural economy. It's the beginning and the end of all that the Lord has done. It is the core of all that He seeks to do to us and through us. John the apostle wrote extensively about love. His gospel is saturated with it and so are his letters. Consider 1 John 4:7-11:

> *Beloved, let us love one another, for love is from God;*
> *and everyone who loves is born of God and knows God.*
> *The one who does not love does not know God, for God is love.*
> *By this the love of God was manifested in us that God has sent*
> *His only begotten Son into the world so that we might live through Him.*

In this is love, not that we loved God, but that He loved us
and sent His Son to be the propitiation for our sins.
Beloved, if God so loved us, we also ought to love one another.

Now that's something to rest in. That's something to set your mind upon! A passage like that has enough truth and wonder in it to keep us worshiping for a lifetime! If we set our mind on the truth about God's love for us and how it was displayed in Jesus, we will be transformed as we experience that love...and then that love will overflow naturally from our lives into the lives of those around us.

> **If we set our mind on the truth about God's love for us and how it was displayed in Jesus, we will be transformed as we experience that love...**

That's pretty amazing when you think about it. He supplies the love we so deeply desire, and in doing so He gives us the ability to pass that love on to others (and even give it back to Him)! His love frees us to freely minister to others. Secure in His love, with our minds set on who we are in Him, we can be free and reckless in our love of others. If we aren't set on Him, we will be concerned only with pleasing others (Galatians 1:10) and our love will always be tentative, calculated, and cold. One of the greatest aspects of living by design is the fact that you are truly free to love God and others.

God's love is also essential to our mission to tell others about His love. The words of the Gospel must be spoken, but the words are confirmed by loving relationships with each other. Our love for each other is a light that confirms to our needy world that we are followers of Christ:

> *By this all men will know that you are My disciples,*
> *if you have love for one another.*
> JOHN 13:35

In fact, the end of all ends is love. It's the standard by which God embraces us, and it's the one thing that He can always offer others through us. He is the source of love and we can rest knowing that He will be the one who loves others through us.

1 John 4:19 says, "We love, because He first loved us." Everything in Scripture climaxes with this love; either God's love for us, or His love overflowing into the lives of

> **Everything in Scripture climaxes with this love; either God's love for us, or His love overflowing into the lives of those around us.**

those around us. In the end, love is the pure essence of all we long for. It is where we find the true joy of life and where captives are set free from the lies of the world.

There should be little surprise, then, that this is where the battle rages the strongest. Satan's deceptive attacks are most devious when he is targeting God's love. Just as the battle for Chichi Jima focused on the messages being sent from the radio stations, the truth about God's love is the focus of all that Satan seeks to distort and deny. But victory, freedom, and an over-flowing sense of mission belong to believer's who have set their minds on the love of God and are resting in Him.

The truth about God's love is worth fighting for in our minds and in our world.

Gracious and Loving God,

I come to you again with empty hands. You alone are the source of all I have, all I am, and all I desire to be and do. Set my mind on you, Lord. Soften my heart that I might know, with my soul as well as my head, that you love me with a love that has no comparison. Set my mind on the things above. Moment-by-moment draw my thoughts to truths about You, heaven, and how you have already seated me with You there.

I love You, Lord, because you first loved me. Today and in the days to come, lead me moment-by-moment and love others through me with the love that only You can give.

Amen.

You are from God, little children,
and have overcome them; because greater is
He who is in you than he who is in the world.
1 JOHN 4:4

PART THREE

A Living and Holy Sacrifice

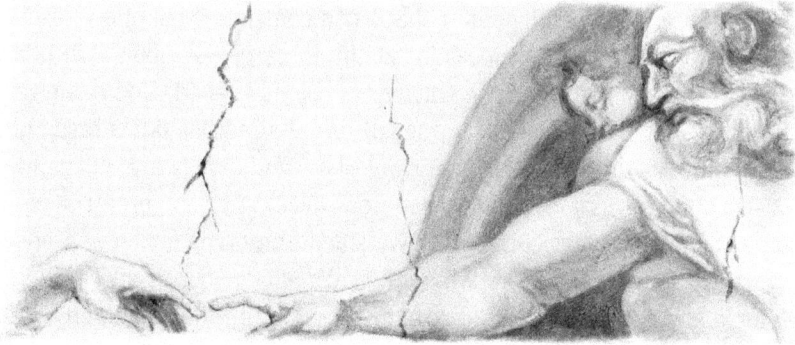

God has given us a great many tools with which to do His will; one of the most amazing is certainly our physical body. It's an absolutely amazing machine and a fantastic display of God's creative design. One of our friends, Bill Gillham, calls the body an "earth suit." I love that word picture. Our flesh and bones are only a temporary container that we have been given for our brief stay on this planet. Soon enough we will eject out of them and move on to better things, but for now the one we have is the only one we will ever get.

He has given us these bodies for several purposes. Romans 12:1 calls us to "present your bodies a living and holy sacrifice, acceptable to God, which is your spiritual service of worship." As long as blood flows in our veins, God calls us to give our bodies over to Him as instruments of praise in everything we do. That's amazing when you think about it. We are to voluntarily offer up our bodies to Him, on His altar, for His work and glorification. That's a wonderful picture, reflecting both our responsibility as the stewards of our bodies and acknowledging God as the ultimate owner of our bodies. Every molecule of muscle and bone is His, yet He has entrusted us to use it as a sacrificial tool for worshiping Him, loving others, and relating to all He has created.

The apostle Paul clearly understood this, and as a result, took a very unique stand toward his body. "I discipline my body and make it my slave," he wrote in 1 Corinthians 9:27. Unfortunately the opposite is true for many of us. In many cases, we become the slaves and our bodies become our masters. Our desires for good looks, our fears of death and illness, and our passions for physical pleasures can dominate our thoughts and our lives. A body that is sick or woefully out of shape can consume most of our resources and our energy as well as block our ability to carry out God's will here on earth. That's backward from the way we've been designed. God has given us these bodies for His purposes for a length of time that He has already determined—and His desire is that they would be used joyfully and efficiently.

Too many of us are wasting away our lives only wishing for a positive change in our physical health when we should be doing something about it as we align and surrender our will with God's will for our lives! Through the scriptures and through a vast amount of research that has emerged over the last two decades, God has revealed a plan that allows us to maximize the days He has given us. That's what the next three chapters are about: developing reasonable, specific, life-enhancing goals that will allow us to get maximum use and pleasure from our "earth suits."

What follows is a concise guide to getting the most out of your body for God's service and worship. The first and most important aspect of protecting our health is to begin resting in the Lord and setting our minds. God's peace will replace anxieties, fears, and worries. You have learned how damaging stress can be in our lives and how it can affect not only our spirit but also our body and soul. I will show you what you can do to make your body as healthy as it can be.

But far more important than what *you do is how you do it.* You must continue to reflect on the motivation of your heart. Please understand this: my fear at this point is that you will leave behind the breakthroughs you've experienced in the last chapters and return to the way you've always approached things in the material world through your own strength. The temptation to return to self-effort and walk in the flesh is never stronger than when we are dealing with issues of the flesh itself, specifically nutrition and exercise. It is critical to understand that you are already totally loved and accepted by God.

It is absolutely essential to understand that "setting the mind," "resting in the Lord," and "walking in the Spirit" were designed by God to permeate every aspect of life. *No matter what you do, this is how it is to be done—with our hearts set on God, what He has done, and who we are in Him.* Each and every act is to be an extension of His life being lived out through us. His moment-by-moment strength and direction propel us into specific actions that are vibrant and useful to the kingdom, reflecting the continually abiding relationship we have with Him. As you choose to focus your heart on God, you'll naturally begin to obey one of the most freeing passages in the Bible, Matthew 6:25, 33:

> *For this reason I say to you, do not be worried about your life,*
> *as to what you will eat or what you will drink; nor for your body,*
> *as to what you will put on. Is not life more than food,*
> *and the body more than clothing? But seek first His Kingdom*
> *and His righteousness, and all these things will be added to you.*

Having a healthy body is not a worthy goal in and of itself. In fact, if we seek that first, we have missed the entire point of our existence. We are called to something infinitely and eternally more important: a vibrant relationship with God that overflows into loving service to others and continual worship of Him as our Creator. The body is simply an earthly tool He has loaned us for that purpose. That truth must always come first. Then (if we are wise) we will seek to make that tool efficient and effective as it can be for that purpose. After all, our body is the temple of the Holy Spirit. Presenting our bodies as a holy and living sacrifice is our spiritual service of worship. God is in control of our health and our life. He knows the very days of our lives. That's what the next part of this book is all about.

In the following chapter we will look at the wonderful advantages we experience when we take control of our bodies and make them our slaves; controlling them, exercising them, and disciplining them for maximum service to us and God's kingdom. In Chapter 8 we will discover how to fuel our bodies with the kinds of foods they were designed to burn. Finally, in Chapter 9 we will look at certain needs that the body has for extra nutrients and vitamins. We will see how adding nutritional supplements to modest exercise and a healthy diet can help protect us from the unusual onslaught of physical attackers in the modern age.

These are all attainable goals; steps that realistically can be done as an extension of our relationship with Him and that also have great benefit to us and to those around us. Because of the body/mind connection, and the integrated nature of our spirit, soul, and body, our goals and the benefits received from them are multifaceted. We will see that: eating and exercise can have great spiritual benefits; that proper nutrition is great for the mind; and why living by spiritual truths impacts everything for the good.

As we proceed, it is critical to continually remember that your value and worth has nothing to do with your performance. It has everything to do with your relationship with the Lord and others. Most importantly, when these goals are pursued in the context of abiding in Christ, resting in the Lord, and setting the mind on the things above, we can have victory over stress and anxiety. Life then becomes an experience of incredible joy and peace as we use our bodies to their fullest potential for their intended purposes of worship, love, and service for as long as God gives us the gift of breath.

> *Lord God,*
> *As we now turn our attention to our bodies, let us never*
> *take our eyes off You. Continually remind us that our flesh*
> *and bones are nothing more than a temporary tool, owned by*
> *You. You created and designed them for worship, service,*
> *and Your great pleasure. We present our bodies to You now*
> *as living sacrifices to be used as You see fit, for as long*
> *or as short as You deem appropriate.*
> *Amen.*

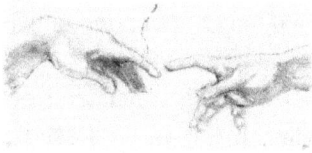

CHAPTER 7

Exercise

Therefore I run in such a way, as not without aim;

I box in such a way, as not beating the air;

but I buffet [discipline] my body and make it my slave

1 CORINTHIANS 9:26-27

We were created for action. The Master Designer has always intended for us to be people of movement—designing us to be continually stretched and challenged. This is true in all areas of life and is obviously true for our bodies. Our "earth suits" were designed to be active on a regular basis. It's mind-boggling to contemplate the physical hardships the body can endure! Consider the challenges faced by ancient nomadic people who crossed great expanses of land. Marvel at the accomplishments of our immigrant forefathers and mothers who survived in the face of drought, rushing rivers, starvation, blizzards, freezing temperatures, wild predators, desert sandstorms, merciless seas, and rugged mountaintops. Through it all the body has been able to survive. Miraculously, when we exercise our bodies properly they actually grow stronger still. The only thing that the body really can't handle is "inactivity."

One of the curses of the modern world, however, is that the body rarely gets to function as it was designed. We have the unfortunate option of living very sedentary, stagnant lives, thanks to cars, escalators, elevators, Internet shopping, fast food, television (remote controls), running water, and even indoor toilets (that now even flush automatically). Major surveys estimate that between 22 percent and 30 percent of U.S. adults participate in no leisure-time physical activity whatsoever (including walking)!

A study published recently in *The New England Journal of Medicine* indicated that physical inactivity might actually be more harmful to our health than other familiar risk factors, such as smoking, hypertension, and cardiovascular disease. The leading author of this study, Jonathan Myers, PhD, stated in the July 2003 issue of *Prevention* magazine, "Our study showed that a person's exercise capacity, measured by their ability to perform on a treadmill, was a more powerful predictor of mortality than all other risk factors."

As a physician, I meet daily with patients immobilized and suffering from the results of arthritis, chronic disease, and excessive weight. I become discouraged by the fact that many of my patients are weakened to the point of being unable to accomplish even simple daily tasks because of their long-term inactivity. Thankfully, most of us have the option to break free and begin using our bodies again—as they were intended—through vibrant, enjoyable, life-giving exercise.

Physical Benefits of Exercise

In the early 1980s, the U.S. Surgeon General issued a statement listing the following health benefits provided by a modest exercise program:

- Weight loss
- Lower blood pressure
- Stronger bones and decreased risk of osteoporosis
- Decreased risk of heart disease
- Improved sensitivity to insulin, which leads to a decreased risk of diabetes
- Increased strength and coordination, which leads to decreased falls and injuries
- Enhanced immune system
- Overall increase in the sense of well-being and greater ability to handle stress

Mental Benefits

Exercise can also do wonders for your mind; it's a great excuse to "get away from it all!" A workout can be a wonderful opportunity to relax your brain, to let your thoughts calm down, and to think about things that have been in the back of your mind for a while. There is a natural relaxation response that follows a good, healthy workout. It is hard to think about the problems facing you at work or at home after a nice, brisk three-mile walk or run.

Exercise is also a potent display of who is in charge of your life. When you push your body, you prove to yourself that your mind is in control, and your flesh is your servant. Most exercise activities are great opportunities to exercise your mind too. Before each work out, choose a passage from the Word, spend a little time contemplating it, and then "set your mind" on that verse throughout the workout, pondering its truth and praying about its application. Pick out some of the passages we studied in the last chapters. As you rest in the Lord, your soul will find peace and strength in the midst of vigorous physical exertion!

Emotional Benefits

Exercise stimulates your body to release natural chemicals called "endorphins". Endorphins attach to special receptor sites in the brain that give you a "natural high." Once you get used to a regular routine of exercise, you will look forward to the feelings you have afterwards. In fact, many people who are struggling with depression, anger, and discouragement find that exercise helps noticeably. Consistent workouts often give them enough relief and hope to move on to better things.

Relational Benefits

Exercise can have a positive impact on relationships too. Time spent in the gym, riding bikes, or hiking are all are prime opportunities to spend quality time with family and friends. ...or workouts can be a great time to be alone. Solitude is rare in life; exercise might be just the right excuse to find it. It may even be an opportunity to shut out the "noise" in our lives, even if it is just for a short period of time. Exercise time can be an opportunity to focus on your relationship with God. It doesn't matter if you are in the mountains or in the weight room.

The benefits of exercise are numerous and can improve every area of our being. It's not just an end in itself; exercise is a means to a lot of wonderful things.

Essential Principles for Successful Exercise

Although exercise can produce magical results, there is no magic involved. We are so fortunate to live in a time when clear and scientific principles are available to the one who wants to improve their fitness. Those who take a haphazard approach to exercise, however, quickly reach a plateau, and the awesome benefits of exercise are minimized. If you follow these general principles for effective exercise, you'll be maximizing the lifetime benefits of a healthy, active life.

1. Check in with a physician

If you are over 40 years of age or have significant risk factors for coronary artery disease (high blood pressure, elevated cholesterol, diabetes), please see your physician before starting any type of exercise program. If you have any musculoskeletal problems (bad back, painful knees, etc.) you should consider having your physician refer you to a physical therapist or chiropractor who can guide you into an exercise program that will not aggravate your underlying condition.

2. Have fun!

Research shows that almost *any* type of exercise is beneficial, so pick something you like! What gets you excited? Fresh air? Friendships? The park? Nature? Gadgets? Speed? Competition? Solitude? Music? Machines? Books? Think about what you like and build your exercise plan around it. I would recommend checking out "the gym scene" before you drop a lot of money on a membership. Gyms might be a great fit for you. You might like the relationships, the mirrors, the music...or, they might make you feel uncomfortable and self-conscious. Most gyms will give you a free trial pass. Try it out before you give them your credit card!

3. Start easy

Whatever you do, take it very easy at first and slowly build up. Your goal is to work up to five balanced workouts per week, each taking about 30 to 40 minutes each. For the first several weeks, just relax and enjoy yourself. Don't overdue it at first! There is no such thing as "fast track fitness" (regardless of what they are trying to sell you on TV). If you've been struggling with weight or have been in poor condition or health for years, it's easy to get excited and determined to get into shape and attempt to do so too quickly.

This is not a race. Each workout is just a short-term goal on the way to a long-term vision. There is no need to get there soon, and trying to do it too fast will lead to burnout, pain, and possible injury that potentially could end your workouts instantly.

4. Gradually push your workouts

It will be amazing how quickly your body will adapt to physical activity if you are wise. When you are feeling stronger and in better condition, you should consider being a little more aggressive with your workouts. Challenging yourself physically will only enhance your health benefits, whether it is allowing your heart to beat a little faster during a burst of aerobic activity or pushing your muscles to near exhaustion during weight resistant exercise. However, remember that *over* exercise can actually be harmful to your health. Simply keep challenging yourself as you see your overall physical strength and cardiovascular condition improving.

5. Adequate rest

Oddly enough, rest is an essential element of successful exercise. Effective exercise actually tears you down. It stresses your body beyond normal limits causing microdamage in your muscles. Your muscles and cardiovascular system heal and become stronger during the rest phase more than during the actual workout! If you are continually working the muscle and cardiovascular system and breaking it down without giving enough time to rest and rebuild, you can actually lose ground. This leads to a common condition called "overtraining," which can lead to fatigue, weakness, decrease in your immune system, and potentially lead to injuries. It's also very discouraging because when you are overtraining, your progress stops even as you are trying harder. Adequate rest for our muscles and bodies is critical for an effective exercise program. Just as resting in the Lord strengthens our soul, it's during rest that muscles grow, heal, and find new strength. For this reason, we recommend no more than five workouts a week, giving your body two days to strengthen and recover.

6. Vary your routine

If you are involved in a weight resistance program, a concept called "muscle memory" will seriously limit any gains you may expect from your workout program. If you simply repeat the same exercise over and over, month after month, the muscle "remembers" and adjusts to the exercise. This will not allow for the breakdown of the muscle that is required for increased strengthening and building up of the muscle.

Mixing up your exercise routine maximizes both effectiveness and enjoyment. If you are a walker, take to the sidewalks, the parks, or to the trails on a regular basis. If you swim, try out different pools or try an open water swim in a lake. In your weight training, it's always a good idea to vary the types of exercises, the kinds of machines you might use, and the amount of weight you lift. No matter what kind of plan you develop, have alternative options handy in case your circumstances change. For instance, if the weather turns bad, you might want to take your walk inside the local mall. (But leave your wallet behind or it could cause stress to your financial health!)

Always remember that any kind of exercise is better than none, so spice it up with some variety!

7. Stay hydrated

Your body needs water. In fact, most of our body and muscle is made up of water. When you exercise it needs even more water than normal. As part of a healthy lifestyle, you will want to start drinking more water throughout your regular day. When you exercise, drink before you get thirsty. If you are planning a long bike ride or a hike on a hot day, drink a couple extra glasses of water several hours before you begin and then keep drinking throughout the activity. Plenty of purified or distilled water ensures that you get the most out of your efforts and prevents dehydration.

8. Make it a priority

Very few of us feel like we have extra time. Even if we had a 48-hour day, we still wouldn't have enough time for everything. That's why we need to take charge and fill our lives with what matters—with what's important. Otherwise, the world and those around us will determine our schedules.

Scheduling our exercise time really isn't that difficult. With our goal of five 30 to 40 minute workouts, we only need two-and-a-half to four hours per week. That's not much considering that the average adult male watches 29 hours of TV and the average female watches 34 hours! If you really can't pry yourself away from the tube, then exercise while you are watching television! Many gyms are equipped with TVs, or you can move your stair-stepper into the living room. All you need to do is make life-giving exercise a priority and other things on the to-do list will begin fit in around it. Be creative and be persistent. Exercise is a very, very good investment of your time.

Creating an Effective, Successful Plan

Your local bookstore undoubtedly has a large section on fitness and exercise. Take a look the next time you are there and you will find nearly every conceivable exercise program. Remember you do not have to be a marathon runner or Mr. America to achieve health benefits from exercise. A simple, consistent exercise program is all that is necessary. Be sure you choose the types of exercise that you will enjoy and look forward to doing.

The Number One Priority: A Solid Aerobic Base

An aerobic exercise causes you to breathe heavier than normal for ten to 30 minutes. Classic examples of aerobic exercise would be walking briskly, jogging, biking, swimming, hiking, tennis, and racquetball; but really, anything will do. Aerobic exercise is the most effective kind of exercise for increasing the health of your heart and lungs and to help reverse insulin resistance, which allows you to decrease your risk of developing heart disease or diabetes.

All types of aerobic exercise have been found to be beneficial in improving insulin sensitivity, especially for those who have been inactive, overweight, and those with type 2 diabetes mellitus. The more aggressive and vigorous the exercise, the greater the effectiveness will be in improving insulin resistance. However, even moderate exercise, is very effective.

> Aerobic exercise is the most effective kind of exercise for increasing the health of your heart and lungs and to help reverse insulin resistance, which allows you to decrease your risk of developing heart disease or diabetes.

Contrary to other diet/exercise programs based on the premise of "calories in, calories out," the reason to exercise is entirely different. The amount of calories used during exercise is insignificant compared to the entire metabolic changes that occur by improving insulin sensitivity. Once you have corrected insulin resistance, your body is finally able to use calories normally and you literally begin releasing fat from those abdominal fat cells. I detail this concept in my book, *Healthy for Life*, (Real Life Press 2005).

Aerobic activities are definitely the place to start for maximum exercise results. Your first goal is to "go aerobic" five times a week, in any kind of activity you desire. Because of the unlimited options available, aerobic exercise can be very enjoyable. Start with very easy, short sessions. (It is more advantageous to go out for a ten-minute walk five times a week than it is to try to walk five miles once a week.) Over the first month or two, build to the point where you are breathing a little harder for 20 to 30 minutes. Once you are able to walk for 30 minutes five times a week, begin pushing yourself by walking more briskly or walking up some hills. To get even more out of your aerobic workout, add several bursts of effort for just a minute or two that take you right to the edge of your capacity; then back off again.

That's really all there is to it. Choose any activities you want from the huge smorgasbord of recreational opportunities, and then go out there and have fun! Don't forget to drink your water and take time off in between sessions for rest.

Building Strength on the Base

While you are building your aerobic base five times a week, you can start adding anaerobic elements to your exercise. Anaerobic exercises create a warm, slow-burning sensation in your muscles and they add wonderful benefits to your aerobic base.

Benefits of Anaerobic Strength Training:
- Increased muscular strength
- Larger muscles that burn more calories
- Increased flexibility and balance
- Decreased risk of heart attack
- Prevention of muscle loss and falls during aging
- Improved bone density and decreased risk of osteoporosis

Essential Principles of Strength Training

1. Resistance.

Resistance can come in many forms. It might be from a coiled spring or an elastic cord. It might be from a metal weight or some sort of mechanical brake. Or it can be as simple as gravity as you do a push-up or sit-up. Even doing heavy yard work or cutting wood will give you some resistance exercise. Regardless of the source, strength training applies resistance to your movements, causing your muscles to work extra hard. Simply "going through the motions" is not going to help much.

A certain amount of stress handled properly is good for the body and it is also good for your muscles. When a muscle is stressed appropriately, there is a break down of the muscle fibers (microdamage), which stimulates muscle growth. Therefore, it is essential that you break down the muscle you are working during your workout and then allow enough time for the muscle to adequately repair itself.

2. "Reps"

When you are exercising a particular muscle, there are two phases of the exercise that must be defined. When you are contracting the muscle, it is called the concentric phase. When you are relaxing the muscle and allowing to return to the starting position, it is called the eccentric phase. When you work out, the concentric phase should last a full two to three seconds. The eccentric phase should take even longer, about three to four seconds. During the eccentric or relaxation phase, the microdamage to the muscle occurs. It is this particular stress on the muscle that stimulates muscle growth. A slow controlled contraction and relaxation of the muscle will not only protect you from injury but also will maximize the effects of your exercise.

Each time you complete one full contraction and one relaxation of the muscle, it's called a "repetition" or a "rep." The number of reps a person performs really varies on what their individual goals really are. However, I personally believe that doing eight to 12 reps for an individual exercise is the safest recommendation. This way you do not have too much or too little weight.

3. Sets

Sets are just clusters of reps with a rest in between. Let's say you do ten reps, three times, with two one-minute rests in between. That would be three "sets."

Understanding how resistance, reps, and sets work together will allow you to customize your strength training to fit your goals. Quite simply, if you want to build big muscles, you want to exercise with more resistance, at fewer reps and sets. If you want to tone your body with muscles that are lean and clean, you will want to have less resistance and do more reps and sets.

Again, for strength training, lift enough weight so that you are not able to exceed 12 reps but can do at least eight reps. If you are doing more than 12 reps, you are essentially doing an aerobic exercise. If you are not able to do eight reps with the weight you have chosen, you have too much resistance and may be vulnerable to injury.

When you are first beginning, it is wise to do between ten and 15 reps. As you improve, you should try to do between eight and 12 reps. Advanced training may involve six to eight reps.

Adjust your resistance so you can do three sets of these reps for each exercise. It is critical that you are just barely able to complete the final rep of each set. In other words, you should be lifting enough weight to completely exhaust and fatigue the muscle you are working somewhere between the eighth and 12th rep, depending on your conditioning level. If you are not able to fatigue the muscle until the 18th rep, you need to increase the amount of resistance (by adding more weight). If you are fatiguing the muscle in the third rep, you are lifting too much weight and you need to lower the resistance (by decreasing the weight).

When you get the hang of this, you might want to inject "supersets" into your routine. In a superset, you exercise different muscles during the same set. (For example, you might do a bicep exercise, then a particular leg exercise, and then an abdominal exercise before taking a rest.) This adds variety and also brings in an element of aerobic exercise (increased pulse rate) into the workout. However, it must be stressed that this should involve working two or three totally different muscle groups to avoid injury.

Keys to Successful Strength Training:
- *Go slow.* Stay in constant control as you carefully move through each rep.
- *Don't fully extend your joints.* Always keep a little bend to avoid the chance of hyperextending or damaging a joint.
- *Stop at the first moment of pain.* Remember, you want to go for the burn, not a break.
- *Start easy and build steadily.* Begin with very easy resistance, always targeting 12 reps and two to three sets for each muscle. Slowly add resistance over a couple of weeks until you are maxed out at the end the third set, feeling a steady burn, and unable to lift any more.
- *Rest.* Take at least a minute in between sets to rest and take a drink of water. Make sure that you take off at least a day in between your strength building exercises for an aerobic workout or a day of complete relaxation.

- *Mix it up.* Your muscles respond best to variety, so as you begin to develop a healthy habit of strength training, you must inject some diversity into your plan. You might want to try a different machine or hold your hands differently. You can alter the position of your body slightly too. Try a few more reps at less resistance or fewer sets at more resistance.
- *Exercise every muscle once a week.* Authorities say that a muscle needs four to seven days to recover from a good strength workout. If you alternate the muscles you exercise, it brings safety and balance to your workouts. I recommend exercising your chest/triceps/abdomen during one work out, legs/shoulders/abdomen the next, and then exercising your back/biceps/abdomen during your final anaerobic strength work out.

A Word about Exercise Equipment.

There are some amazing machines that have been invented to help you exercise. Some work great, some are okay, and many are next to worthless. I recommend starting simply, inexpensively, and then adding equipment as your plan evolves.

It's actually possible to start your strength training without any equipment at all! I call it the "Weightless Workout." It uses gravity as your only resistance and makes use of simple exercises such as push-ups, sit-ups, chair dips, knee bends, wall sits, and stair climbing to give you an effective anaerobic workout.

If you decide to head to the gym, you will find everything you need there, and usually pretty good advice from the trainers.

If you want to begin creating your own home gym, start simply with some dumbbells, which can be bought for 50 cents a pound at most sports stores. Don't buy anything massive or expensive until you are absolutely sure it fits your taste—and check the newspaper before buying new. The classifieds are full of people trying to get rid of "barely used" exercise equipment that they bought on a whim as part of their last New Year's resolution.

Putting It All Together.

Your weekly plan will reflect your priorities, your goals, and your preferences. It will reasonably fit into your schedule and build slowly over time until you have an awesome, life-enhancing new experience as a regular part of your life.

In its simplest form your weekly plan will include:
- Five aerobic activities that get you breathing fairly hard for at least 30 minutes.
- Two or three strength building workouts that get your major muscles burning once a week. (This can actually be a part of your aerobic exercise or be done at the beginning or end of an aerobic workout.)

A typical, balanced plan might look something like this:

Sunday:	Rest Day
Monday:	Aerobic Activity #1: Morning bike ride
	Strength Building #1: Chest/triceps/abdomen
Tuesday:	Aerobic Activity #2: A rigorous evening hike with friends and family
Wednesday:	Aerobic Activity #3: Jog in the park during lunch
Thursday:	Aerobic Activity #4: Treadmill
	Strength Building #2: Legs/shoulders
Friday:	Rest day
Saturday:	Aerobic Activity #5: Stationary bike while watching TV or reading a book
	Strength Building #3: Back/biceps

God created your incredible body to be a vibrant, submissive tool for His work. It is an instrument of praise, a tool for service, and a loudspeaker for truth. As you give your body regular exercise, every area of your life is enhanced: the physical, emotional, relational, mental, and even the spiritual. The more opportunity you give your body to move, the more every area of your life will be strengthened to carry out His will.

Why not look at your schedule right now and plan your aerobic activities for this week? Better yet, why don't you dust off your bike right now and go for a quick ride? You've got nothing to loose (except maybe some extra pounds!) and everything to gain.

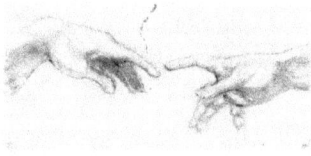

CHAPTER 8

Healthy Diet

All things are lawful for me, but not all things are profitable.
All things are lawful for me, but I will not be
mastered by anything. Food is for the stomach and the stomach
is for food, but God will do away with both of them.

1 CORINTHIANS 6:12-13

The God of the universe satisfies. The roots of our deepest hungers are planted in a God-created desire to find fulfillment in Him. He created our souls to hunger and thirst for righteousness, and to long for Him as a deer pants for water (Psalm 42:1). God created us to find satisfaction in Him and Him alone, so that He alone would get the glory and praise, for truly He alone is worthy (Psalm 16).

In the same way, He created our bodies to find satisfaction in certain kinds of foods that give energy, health, and protection to our "earth suits"— suits that are really only temporary tools for service and worship during our brief stay on this planet. The foods we eat supply the carbohydrates, proteins, fats, vitamins, minerals, and antioxidants that our bodies need to function properly. Just as we must feed our spirit and soul as we learn to "abide in Christ," "rest in the Lord," and "set our mind," so we need to learn how to nourish our physical bodies properly.

Your body is important! It's the only one you've got and the only one you will get on this planet. But as Paul notes in 1 Corinthians 6:19-20, there is another profound and powerful reason God created your body:

Your body is important! It's the only one you've got and the only one you will get on this planet.

Or do you not know that your body is a temple
of the Holy Spirit who is in you, whom you have from God,
and that you are not your own? For you have been bought
with a price: therefore glorify God in your body.

How many of us truly glorify God *in our bodies?* How many of us even think about glorifying God *in our bodies?* Most of us don't even give it a second thought! How you take care of your body and what types of food and drink you put into your body reflect your worship of the living and holy God that lives within you!

Therefore I urge you, brethren, by the mercies of God,
to present your bodies a living and holy sacrifice, acceptable to God,
which is your spiritual service of worship.
ROMANS 12:1

What an interesting link this passage makes regarding the body/soul/spirit design. This command to present your body as a living and holy sacrifice to the Lord is truly an act of "spiritual" worship… and it is an act of your *will.*

If you humble yourself and surrender your will to God's truth, you will be walking in the Spirit and you will not carry out the deeds of the flesh. However, if we walk according to the flesh, we carry out the deeds of the flesh. I personally feel true believers struggle more with the desires of the flesh when it comes to food than with any other aspect of their faith. We all realize that drunkenness, adultery, pornography, immorality, and carousing are signs of walking in the flesh. However, most of us do not realize that there is an addictive side to food that creates a powerful bondage in the flesh.

Christians must realize and respect the fact that our body is now the temple of the Holy Spirit. God has given us our physical bodies to use to carry out His will in this world. Not only can poor eating habits create bondage but also they can destroy our health and seriously hinder our souls.

Over 65 percent of adults and over 30 percent of children in the United States are either overweight or obese. The Center for Disease Control (CDC) projects those Caucasian children born after the year 2000 have over a 30 percent risk of developing diabetes sometime during their lifetime. (The rate is nearly 50 percent for African American, Hispanic, and Native American children). This is a *major* concern: diabetes is the leading cause of blindness, kidney failure, amputations, and neuropathy, and over 80 percent of diabetics will die prematurely due to a cardiovascular event such as a heart attack or stroke. I believe that these statistics may be even *worse* for believers in Christ. We certainly perish for lack of knowledge. The truth is that many of us carry excess weight, do not exercise like we should, and are consuming foods that are far, far from what God designed our bodies to use. Then when our health finally fails, we turn to God for a miracle.

Within certain constraints, the Christian is free to eat or do whatever he or she chooses:

I personally feel true believers struggle more with the desires of the flesh when it comes to food than with any other aspect of their faith.

> *I know and am convinced in the Lord Jesus*
> *that nothing is unclean in itself; but to him who*
> *thinks anything to be unclean, to him it is unclean.*
> ROMANS 14:14

> *For you were called to freedom, brethren;*
> *only do not turn your freedom into an opportunity for the flesh,*
> *but through love serve one another.*
> GALATIANS 5:13

> *"Surely not, Lord!" Peter replied. "I have never eaten*
> *anything impure or unclean." The voice spoke to him a second time,*
> *"Do not call anything impure that God has made clean."*
> ACTS 10:14-15

Recently, Christians have been giving more attention to what should or should not be eaten. Many books and many Christian television programs have focused on "How Would Jesus Eat?," "The Maker's Diet," and "Body by God," to name a few. A proper biblical mindset, however, is a vital prerequisite to any kind of "diet." Scripture is very clear in Romans 14:14 that nothing is unclean and that God's grace has freed us from the bondage of legalism (even when it comes to food!). We are not to judge one another in the body of Christ and love for one another is the most important concern. The kingdom of God is NOT about eating and drinking, but righteousness and peace and joy in the Holy Spirit (Romans 14:17). At the same time, however, Paul warns us not to turn our freedom into an opportunity for the flesh (Galatians 5:13). Not everything is in our best interest, especially when it comes to how we choose to nourish our bodies!

Our physical bodies have been designed by God to need certain fuels to be able to function at optimal levels. This includes a balance of good carbohydrates, good proteins, and good fats combined with a modest exercise program and now in this modern day world nutritional supplementation. This information has been recorded in detail in my books, *What Your Doctor Doesn't Know about Nutritional Medicine* (Thomas Nelson 2002) and *Healthy for Life* (Real Life Press 2005). If you would like to learn more details about this subject, I would certainly refer you to these books.

The Root Problem: High-glycemic Carbohydrates

Our bodies need carbohydrates. Don't get caught up in the "low-carb craze" that is taking over the U.S. and Canada. God designed our bodies to need and desire carbohydrates as its number one fuel source. Carbohydrates provide the fuel that the body and the brain desire, and good carbohydrates contain the vitamins, minerals, and antioxidants that our bodies need. We have to learn, however, that there are good carbohydrates and there are bad carbohydrates. The root issue is the fact that certain carbohydrates are converted unnaturally fast into blood sugar within our bodies. When these foods are consumed on a regular basis, the body is set on a roller-coaster ride of rising and falling blood sugar levels that God never designed it to cope with...and the results are often *deadly*.

For over a century now, the medical community has believed that the ability of the body to absorb carbohydrates (and thus raise blood sugar levels) has been based on a concept of "simple sugar" versus "complex carbohydrates." Since carbohydrates are long chains of sugar, this theory is based on the belief that shorter sugar chains are absorbed more quickly. Simple sugars, like table sugar, were felt to be absorbed much quicker than foods such as white bread, which is a complex carbohydrate. This is why the base of the USDA food pyramid (even the new one) is made up of bread, cereals, rice, and potatoes and the peak of the food pyramid is made up of primarily sweets and sugar.

In 1981, Dr. David Jenkins from the University of Toronto took another look at this theory and put it to the test. His research was simple. He tested how quickly blood sugar levels rose after eating a particular carbohydrate, and compared it to a control food, which was usually glucose. He gave glucose a glycemic index of 100, since glucose is what all carbohydrates become in the blood stream when it is broken down by the body. The test was simple, but the results were very, very surprising. (See Table 1.)

TABLE 1
Glycemic Index and Glycemic Load of Some Common Foods

	GLYCEMIC INDEX	GLYCEMIC LOAD
Glucose	100	10
Fructose (fruit sugar)	19	6
Sucrose (table sugar)	61	6
Bakery Goods		
Angel food cake	67	19
Croissant	67	17
Doughnut, cake	76	17
Muffin, bran	60	15
Vegetables		
Carrots	49	2.4
Peas	48	3
Corn, sweet	54	9
Fruits		
Apple	38	6
Cherry	22	3
Orange	42	5
Peach	28	4

	GLYCEMIC INDEX	GLYCEMIC LOAD
Legumes		
Beans, kidney	28	7
Beans, black	20	5
Breads		
Bagel, white	72	25
Bread, white	70	10
Bread, whole wheat flour	71	8
Potato		
Baked, white	85	26
Instant, mashed	85	17
Mashed potato	92	18

Surprisingly, many complex carbohydrates (such as white bread, rice, potatoes, and cereals) actually spiked blood sugar faster than raw table sugar! A baked potato, which is a complex carbohydrate, had a glycemic index of 85 while table sugar or sucrose had a glycemic index of only 61. This went against all the conventional wisdom of the past century! A carbohydrate was no longer just a carbohydrate. You now had to consider the glycemic index of a carbohydrate before you would know how it was going to affect the body.

Further research brought up another concept called "glycemic load." Glycemic load not only takes into account the glycemic index but also how many calories that carbohydrate contains. The concept of glycemic load provides a much better picture of one's response to a particular food. A food such as cooked carrots has a moderate glycemic index of 49 while its glycemic load is very low at 2.4 (Any glycemic load less than ten is low). This means that you basically can't eat enough carrots to spike your blood sugar. However, potatoes have both a high glycemic index and a high glycemic load, which will significantly spike your blood sugar.

Determining the Glycemic Load

Glycemic load= (Glycemic Index x Grams of Carbohydrate) divided by 100

Spaghetti: 1 cup of cooked spaghetti has a Glycemic Index of 41 and contains 52 grams of carbohydrate.

Glycemic Load: (41x52) divided by 100 = 21

Carrots: Glycemic index is 49 and the average serving contains an average of 5 grams of carbohydrates per serving.

Glycemic Load: (49 x 5) divided by 100 = 2.4

This example illustrates that glycemic index is only one aspect in choosing quality carbohydrates. If you were to consider only the glycemic index, spaghetti looks like a better choice than carrots. However, when you look at the grams of carbohydrates you are consuming with one serving (2 ounces or 1/2 cup) of spaghetti (52 grams) compared with the amount of carbohydrates consumed with an average serving of carrots (5 grams), it becomes apparent that the spaghetti is going to create a greater rise in our blood sugar—especially when you consider that the average amount of pasta served in an Italian restaurant today is equal to eight to ten servings! See Table 1 to see the glycemic load of some common foods or the list of foods in the resource pages.

Events Following a High-Glycemic Meal or Snack

The body needs to control blood sugar in a very narrow range. Our brain or mind thinks on blood sugar. If our blood sugar gets too high or too low, it can cause serious problems for the body and soul. When you consume a high-glycemic meal such as instant oatmeal or a bagel, your blood sugar rises very rapidly. This rapidly rising blood sugar stimulates the release of insulin. Insulin's job is to control blood sugar by driving blood sugar into the cell either to be utilized as energy or stored as glycogen or fat. The major problem with spiking your blood sugar is that you actually *over* stimulate the release of insulin. This causes the blood sugar to go down almost as fast as it went up, usually dropping the blood sugar into the hypoglycemic or low blood sugar range.

If blood sugar was allowed to continue to fall, you not only could experience a shaky weakness but also you can become mentally confused, possibly have a seizure, or even go into a coma. However, the low blood

So not only does physical and emotional stress increase the amount of stress hormones you have in your bloodstream, but *the way you eat has a tremendous effect on stress hormone levels as well!*

sugar stimulates the release of the stress hormones such as adrenaline and cortisol that we talked about in chapter 2. These hormones drive the blood sugar back up to normal...but now you have elevated levels of these stress hormones in your blood stream. So not only does physical and emotional stress increase the amount of stress hormones you have in your bloodstream, *but the way you eat has a tremendous effect on stress hormone levels as well!*

Worse yet, the elevated stress hormones in your blood cause an *uncontrollable* hunger. Your body tells you that you must eat again (and usually you crave another high-glycemic meal)...and the vicious cycle starts all over again.

Usually this has been labeled "cravings" or "emotional eating" but it is really an irresistible hunger triggered by spiking your blood sugar and consequently stimulating the release of stress hormones as your blood sugar drops due to excessive insulin release. I refer to this as a "Carbohydrate Addiction," and it is as strong an addiction as caffeine, nicotine, alcohol, and even most drugs.

Eighty-five to 90 percent of the carbohydrates that we are presently consuming in this country are either highly processed or high-glycemic. That's one of the main reasons we are facing the obesity and diabetic epidemic today. Yes, some foods addict and some foods satisfy, and your choice between these foods has life-impacting implications.

Insulin Resistance—the Metabolic Syndrome

After years of repeatedly spiking blood sugar levels, the cells of the body become less and less sensitive to insulin. When this happens, the body compensates by making more and more insulin. As the blood insulin levels begin to rise, the body "tips over" into an abnormal state called "the metabolic syndrome." The "metabolic syndrome" is a constellation of problems caused by the increasing levels of insulin in your body and include high blood pressure, central weight gain, and elevated cholesterol and triglyceride levels. These factors significantly increase the risk of heart disease and diabetes. Arteries also begin aging much faster than they should. When we live outside of God's design, the consequences can be fatal.

Central Obesity and Diabetes

People who develop the metabolic syndrome gain a significant amount of weight around their middle. Medical research is now showing us that muscle cells become insulin resistant first. Muscle normally burns up 85 to 90 percent of calories from any meal or snack, but when muscle becomes insulin resistant, many of these calories are diverted to the fat cells of the abdomen. You now have the worst possible situation: Your muscles are no longer able to utilize the calories you consume normally and your blood insulin levels are high. In this situation a calorie is no longer a calorie. You simply start putting on an unusual amount of weight around your middle.

Nearly 25 percent of the adult population and many of our children already have full-blown insulin resistance and another 25 percent are on their way to developing it. If you have insulin resistance, you cannot lose weight. You hold on to fat like a sponge holds on to water. No matter what you try to do you cannot lose weight effectively. But that is a minor problem compared to what lies ahead: In another ten to 15 years your body will not be able to keep making all that insulin, and eventually your insulin levels begin to drop. When that happens, your blood sugars will begin to rise uncontrollably... and you'll find yourself with type 2 or adult-onset diabetes mellitus.

Please, please understand what I'm saying now: *You have the freedom to eat whatever you choose, but when you choose to continually eat things that your body was not designed for, there will be consequences.* The processes I've described above are fascinating and intriguing and a definite tribute to the creativity of the Master Designer. But the fact is that our bodies (as well as our spirits and souls) were designed to function within limited parameters.

The answer to the diet dilemma is to develop healthy lifestyles that improve insulin sensitivity and prevent the metabolic syndrome. If you already have the metabolic syndrome, exercise, a proper diet, and nutritional supplements allow you to "tip back" into a normal metabolic state and reverse this insulin resistance. The consequence of living by design is an improved chance to prevent heart disease and diabetes and have permanent weight loss as a positive side effect.

Events Following a Low-Glycemic Meal or Snack

When you eat a low-glycemic meal or snack that does not spike your blood sugar, blood sugar rises slowly. The release of insulin is not over stimulated. Consequently, blood sugar levels do not fall into the low blood sugar range and stress hormones are not released. You are much more satisfied, the satisfaction lasts for a longer period of time, and you do not set off this uncontrollable hunger. Insulin levels begin to fall and you become much more sensitive to your own insulin.

Learning to eat meals that provide healthy nutrients and that do not spike blood sugar levels goes a long way in helping you protect your health and the temple of the Holy Spirit.

Carbohydrates that Satisfy and Carbohydrates that Addict

Certain carbohydrates satisfy and certain carbohydrates lead to a true carbohydrate addiction. Whole fruits, whole vegetables, legumes, nuts, and whole grains are generally low to moderate in their glycemic index and therefore will not spike your blood sugar or set off uncontrollable hunger. (The exception is the white potato, which is naturally very high-glycemic.)

In general the more man processes the food, the higher its glycemic index and the easier it is for the body to absorb the sugars and spike our blood sugar. So go for less processing. For example, the apple is better than applesauce. The applesauce is better than the apple juice. The apple juice is better than the sweetened apple juice. If you take whole oats and soak them overnight and then cook and eat them in the morning, they are low-glycemic. If you have slow-cooked rolled oats for breakfast, they have a moderate glycemic index. Instant oatmeal (as you should now suspect) is *very* high-glycemic.

God has created a tremendous variety of food that is able to help nourish our bodies and provide most of the macro- and micronutrients our bodies require. Just think about all of the different fruits and vegetables that are available as you walk around the *outside* aisles of your local grocery store! Food that is fresh, natural, and in its original state (what some refer to as whole food) is ideal for the body. Apples, pears, beans, legumes, nuts, broccoli, cauliflower, carrots, whole grains are excellent choices... and the list goes on and on. These foods satisfy and provide the kinds of nutrients our bodies need.

Eating a healthy diet is not really that difficult. You simply have to stay on the outside of your grocery store and avoid going into those middle aisles!

As you begin to enter the *inside* aisles of grocery stores, you begin to encounter a host of processed foods that have been canned, boxed, and wrapped. These foods have been processed to provide you instant meals, tasty pastries, refined cereals and grains, refined bread, chips, crackers, and "snack" foods. Eating a healthy diet is not really that difficult. You simply have to stay on the outside of your grocery store and avoid going into those middle aisles!

If you have gone to a party recently where they have a table of hors d'oeuvres, you will usually find on one end the potato chips, tortilla chips, corn chips, and dip. On the other end of the table you find the apples, pears, bananas, and melon. What is the host or hostess generally doing? Most often they are filling up the chip bowels and the fruit is usually lasting much longer. Well, have you ever stopped to think about why we tend to continue eating the chips? Is it because this is the good food and the fruit is not? Is it because apples or bananas taste bad? The difference is the fact that the chips addict and the fruit satisfies.

I certainly love bananas, however, usually I can't eat more than one. Have you ever eaten five apples or bananas in a row? But when was the last time you were served a large order of French fries and then did not eat them all, even if you "Supersized" them? I certainly can't stop eating them. There is definitely truth behind the fact that you can't have just one Lay's potato chip.

In the resource section of this book, I have listed the most common carbohydrates. They are listed in three categories (desirable, moderately desirable, and least desirable). I have taken into account the nutritional quality of the carbohydrate, its glycemic index, and its glycemic load. It is a great resource, however, common sense tells you that food that is eaten in its most natural state and not overcooked is better for you. People who do eat their eight to 12 servings of fruits and vegetables daily significantly decrease their risk of heart disease, cancer, diabetes, and Alzheimer's dementia. These are the foods that also contain great antioxidants and their supporting nutrients. In fact, these foods should make the base of your food pyramid. (See Figure 1)

People who do eat their eight to 12 servings of fruits and vegetables daily significantly decrease their risk of heart disease, cancer, diabetes, and Alzheimer's dementia.

Good Fats and Bad Fats

Fat is the second important macronutrient that we need to discuss. Fats are essential to our health. They are used by our bodies to build cell membranes, brain cells, nerves, and many of our hormones. For the last 40 years we've been advised to decrease our consumption of fat at all cost. But again,

FIGURE 1
Living by Design Food Pyramid

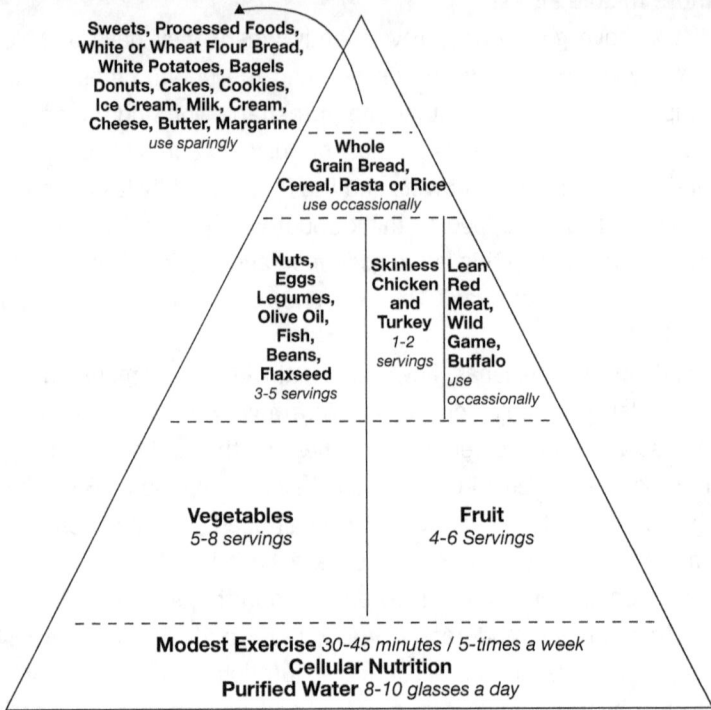

Sweets, Processed Foods,
White or Wheat Flour Bread,
White Potatoes, Bagels
Donuts, Cakes, Cookies,
Ice Cream, Milk, Cream,
Cheese, Butter, Margarine
use sparingly

Whole
Grain Bread,
Cereal, Pasta or Rice
use occassionally

Nuts,
Eggs
Legumes,
Olive Oil,
Fish,
Beans,
Flaxseed
3-5 servings

Skinless
Chicken
and
Turkey
*1-2
servings*

Lean
Red
Meat,
Wild
Game,
Buffalo
*use
occassionally*

Vegetables
5-8 servings

Fruit
4-6 Servings

Modest Exercise *30-45 minutes / 5-times a week*
Cellular Nutrition
Purified Water *8-10 glasses a day*

the key to fueling your body isn't necessarily in the *quantity* of fat you consume or even in the amount of *calories* in the fat you consume. The important thing is the *kinds* of fat you eat. We now know that there are definitely good fats and there are bad fats. Eating good fats actually decreases the levels of our bad cholesterol. Eating good fats even helps you lose fat! (That goes against conventional wisdom, of course, but the medical evidence now strongly supports this new position.) Let's take a look and the different kinds of fats, where they are found, and how to get them in proper balance.

Saturated Fats

Saturated fats are the most consumed fat in the Western world. They are found in all red meats, white meats, and dairy products. Unfortunately they aren't good to have around. When they are burned as fuel, saturated fats breakdown into "acetate fragments" which the liver can quickly convert into cholesterol.

Cholesterol

Cholesterol is a very important fat in several respects. It is needed for the production of vital hormones such as testosterone, estrogen, and cortisol. It is required for the production of bile acids and cell membranes. Of the two major types of cholesterol, HDL is considered "good" and LDL is considered "bad." Yet over the last two decades, *all* cholesterol has gotten a bad reputation. Cholesterol is found in the hardened plaque within the arteries of those with heart disease, so we've been taught to reduce it in our diets. Studies are now showing, however, that decreasing the amount of cholesterol in the *diet* has very little effect on lowering cholesterol levels in the *blood*. High consumption of saturated fats and high-glycemic carbohydrates is what raises our blood cholesterol levels. *By focusing on good fats and carbohydrates with a low-glycemic index and load, people with high cholesterol levels can potentially significantly lower their cholesterol levels.*

Trans-fats

Trans-fats are "the bad boys of fat" and are normally considered to be the worst fats you can put in your body. Because of their negative impact on health, they have been totally banned in Europe. Most trans-fats started out as good fats from vegetable oils that were heated, hydrogenated, or partially hydrogenated and now are some of the worst fats you can consume. (It's ironic that margarine, which has been marketed as a healthy alternative to butter, is loaded with trans-fats.) The best way to stay out of trouble is to avoid these guys. Stay away from highly processed foods and margarine, and check the labels for anything that mentions "trans-fat" or "partially hydrogenated fat."

Monosaturated Fat

Monosaturated fats are found in olives, olive oil, almonds, peanuts, pistachios, pecans, canola oil, avocados, hazelnuts, cashews, and macadamia nuts. These fats are your friends and are considered the good fats. They actually lower levels of bad LDL cholesterol and raise the levels of the good HDL cholesterol. They help lower inflammation in the arteries and decrease the risk of heart disease. Interestingly, monosaturated fats are abundant in olive oil and that may explain the lower incidence of heart disease and breast cancer in the Mediterranean population.

The Mediterranean diet has received a significant amount of attention by the medical community during the past few years. Mediterranean people consume 40 percent of their calories in fat (primarily monosaturated fat from olive oil) and still have a very low incidence of cardiovascular disease. Olive oil is abundant in oleic acid and is felt to be a contributing factor (along with its phenols) for the low incidence of heart disease and several cancers among the Mediterranean population. The consumption of olive oil has been specifically associated with a marked decreased risk of breast cancer.

Polyunsaturated Fats

These fats are known as "essential fatty acids" because, just as their name implies, they are essential to the body. The body is not able to make them on its own, so we must get them from our diets. The two kinds to be concerned about are the omega-6 and the omega-3 fatty acids. Omega-6 is found in meats, dairy products, and processed foods. Omega-3 fats are found in flax seed, almonds, soybean oil, walnuts, range-fed chicken eggs, and cold-water fish.

The problem is one of balance. God designed the body to need about two times more omega-6 than omega-3, but in the Western world, we consume about 20 to 30 times more omega-6 than we do omega-3 essential fats. Since Omega-6 produces inflammatory products in the body and omega-3 produces anti-inflammatory products, this imbalance is something to be concerned about. Our bodies simply have too much inflammation. We need to be eating more foods containing omega-3 fats or supplementing our diet with cold-pressed flax seed or filtered fish oil capsules to increase our intake of omega-3 to reduce this inflammation and bring inflammation back into balance.

Fats are an essential aspect of a healthy diet. You should set a goal to begin replacing the bad fat in your diet with the good fat. Therefore, as you decrease your intake of saturated and trans-fats, you should be increasing your intake of monosaturated fat and the omega-3 essential fats.

Power Proteins

Like good carbs and good fats, protein is vital for our existence. Protein is more plentiful than any other substance in the human body except water. Muscles, skin, hair, eyes, and nails are made mostly from protein. It is the building block of the enzymes that make up the core of the immune system. It is also important for the rebuilding of muscles in people like you, who are exercising regularly. Protein breaks down much more slowly than most carbohydrates, smoothing out blood sugar levels. It also stimulates the release of a hormone called cholecystokinin (CCK), which regulates digestion and curbs hunger.

People who eat good proteins tend to eat smaller meals and feel more lasting satisfaction from them. Proteins in a meal or snack also stimulate the release of glucagon, our "fat releasing" hormone. All these aspects of proteins have the effect of increasing insulin sensitivity. Eating quality carbohydrates, fats, and proteins can significantly help to reverse insulin resistance and reduce our chances of developing high blood pressure, high cholesterol and triglyceride levels, heart disease, and diabetes. It also allows the body to "tip back" into a normal metabolic state where the body releases unwanted fat from our midsection.

Protein is protein, but it comes in many different kinds of foods. Most of the proteins we eat in this country come from red meats and dairy products and this has given protein a bad name, since these foods are also loaded with saturated fats. Vegetable proteins contain less fat, but they may lack some of the essential amino acids that the body needs to make its own proteins. However, when you combine a broad base of vegetables and vegetable proteins, the body can get all the essential proteins it needs.

By far the best sources of protein are vegetable proteins such as nuts, beans, soy, and legumes. Cold-water fish like salmon, mackerel, trout, tuna, and sardines are the next best source of protein because they also contain the good omega-3 essential fats. The next best protein source is fowl such as chicken and turkey. Even though they contain saturated fat, the fat is on the outside of the bird under the skin and not marbled into the meat. (It's not a bad idea to trim this off and eat the skinless fowl.)

The least desirable sources of protein come from red meats and dairy products. When selecting red meats, always choose the leanest meat you can afford. The best choices are wild game, buffalo, and organically raised grass-fed cattle. When you eat dairy products be sure that they are low-fat or nonfat dairy products. One of the greatest sources of saturated fat in the American diet comes from butter fat. Skimmed milk, low-fat cottage cheese, low-fat and low-sugar yogurt, along with low-fat cheeses are your best option. Getting a non-hydrogenated vegetable spread such as Smart Balance is also a good idea. These contain the good fats that our bodies need.

Pulling It All Together: The Living by Design Food Pyramid

You remember the old USDA food pyramid. It's in nearly every kid's health textbook and has been the core of our diets for decades. Obviously it isn't working now and never really did. The old USDA food pyramid ignores the kinds of foods that we were designed to eat before the age of highly processed foods. Recently the pyramid has been modified, but it still has at its base that 50% of the grains be highly refined and processed grains, breads, and cereals—which have a higher glycemic index than sugar! (These foods should have been placed at the very tip of the pyramid, since they are worse than candy.) Neither of the USDA food pyramids reflects the best and most resent medical research. With no regrets, the old pyramid deserves to be filed away as history.

In its place, we offer you the Eating by Design Food Pyramid. It is built on the best and most recent revelations in modern medicine; revelations that tell us that God's design hasn't changed since the dawn of creation, and that simple adjustments to our diets will result in major health benefits for our bodies and our souls. *Be encouraged, eating by design is not based on saying "no" but on saying "yes!" While typical diets deny, God's ways always satisfy. In fact, we recommend that you eat more often than you probably do now.* Adding quality snacks throughout the day curbs your hunger, keeps your energy levels high, and minimizes the quantities of food that you will eat during main meals. That's always preferable to stuffing yourself a couple of times a day.

Reflecting what we now know to be true through the glycemic index and thousands of other scientific nutritional studies, the foundation of the pyramid is built on high quality, low-glycemic carbohydrates. Eating eight to 12 servings of whole fruits and vegetables will probably be the landmark change in your diet, breaking you of the slavery of high-glycemic carbohydrates and fueling your body for freedom. High quality proteins and fats make up the next level, containing many of the essential fats and nutrients that make our bodies strong and resistant to disease.

Whole grains and cereals make up the next level. These aren't the highly processed grains that have been drained of their nutrients, but quality kinds of foods that not only don't spike your blood sugar but also retain important vitamins and fiber. Whole grains are important aspects of a healthy diet, however, we do not need to be eating a large quantity of these carbohydrates.

The top of the pyramid represents the most highly processed, high-glycemic carbohydrates. These should be minimized as much as possible and replaced by the quality, low-glycemic carbohydrates at the foundation of the pyramid.

Always remember that eating the *kinds* of foods that give you high quality carbohydrates, fats, and proteins is more important than the *quantity* you eat and it's even more important than the amount of *calories* you eat. When you are eating by design, you leave a meal satisfied—not hungry and not stuffed. You should never go hungry or miss any meals unless you are involved in fasting and prayer.

It is also critical to remember to drink plenty of purified water. Water is critical for the body and your health. Consuming 8 to ten glasses of purified water daily is a very important aspect of health. This can most easily be accomplished by having a glass of purified water available at all times. This allows you to be drinking water throughout the day so you can remain well hydrated. Consuming a large amount of coffee, sodas, diet sodas, and various other sweetened drinks is not only unhealthy but also can cause dehydration because of their diuretic affect. Purified water would be considered water that has been treated by reverse osmosis, high-quality filtration, or distilled.

Energizing your body with the right kinds of carbohydrates, fats, and proteins is one of the essential keys to living by design, and the rewards reach beyond your body and into your very soul and mind.

Energizing your body with the right kinds of carbohydrates, fats, and proteins is one of the essential keys to living by design, and the rewards reach beyond your body and into your very soul and mind. If you are wrestling with some unwanted weight or you have evidence of insulin resistance, combine this healthy diet with a modest exercise program and nutritional supplementation. You will be able to achieve tremendous health benefits and you also lose weight permanently.

The Choice Is Yours

Eating by design is simple, it's powerful, and it's definitely doable. Now you know what kinds of foods will fuel your body for freedom. It's up to you to make the choice to go for it. It's the choice that will lead to a life that is as healthy as can be and give you the energy to seek first the kingdom of God with all your physical strength.

Please, please know, however, that if you give this your best effort, you are doomed to failure. You are not designed to do this on your own. *The crippling effects of self-effort are never more obvious than they are when it comes to traditional diets.* The legalism and self-consciousness that are at the foundation of most plans simply do not work.

Eating by design really isn't about food and it isn't about results. Those are nice benefits when we take our focus off of food and off our bodies and focus on our real goal of resting in the Lord and setting our minds on Him. Jesus wants to dine with you. Most of us have asked Him into our lives, but when it comes time for a meal or a snack, we leave Him in the living room as we head to the kitchen.

> Get this: Jesus desires to have a personal, passionate, and integrated relationship with you in all areas of life—and that specifically includes eating together!

Get this: Jesus desires to have a personal, passionate, and integrated relationship with you in all areas of life—and that specifically includes eating together! As the temple of the Holy Spirit, God dwells inside you and never leaves you. God wants your union together to be evident as the two of you go to the grocery store and decide together what to buy that day. He is available for casual conversation in the kitchen as you prepare your meals. When you rest in the Lord, each meal or snack has the potential to be an intimate candlelit dinner between the two of you, and it is something to be shared with others who are around you. Jesus has invited Himself over for dinner. Will you let Him in?

Lord of the Harvest,

I desire to see my body used to bring You maximum glory. My hope is to fuel it with the things you designed it to burn. But God, I know that I cannot and should not try to do this on my own. I surrender it all to You right now.

I thank You for my body, just as it is. Every single cell of it reflects Your perfect provision for me at this very moment and is a gift from You. Take my mind off my body. Free me from my obsession with its performance and appearance. I choose to not weigh it or measure it. My value and worth are based in what You have done to me and who I am as Your child. I'm asking You to dominate my thoughts, taking the focus off of me and what I eat. I invite You as the honored guest at every meal or snack I eat.

By Your wisdom, let's choose together the things to put in this body. By Your strength, I ask that Your discipline would be my discipline. By Your constant presence in my life, I ask that You would transform meals into a wonderful time of fellowship and worship that we can share together and with those around us. Thank You for the freedom I have in You. Fuel my body in a way that frees me to serve You and worship You like never before.

Amen.

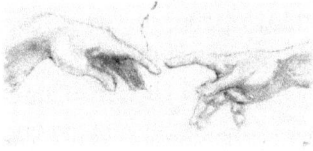

CHAPTER 9

Optimizing God's Defenses: Nutritional Supplements

Grace and peace be multiplied to you in the knowledge of God

and of Jesus our Lord; seeing that His divine power

has granted to us everything pertaining to life...

2 PETER 1:2-3

The study of the human body is a fascinating and intriguing endeavor. If you are a student of the natural sciences, or even have a casual interest in how biology works, you understand that it is an inexhaustible field of interest. An entire universe of activity continually moves within every cell in our body. Actually, that is an understatement! The ballet of molecules and cells that dance with such beauty and precision within us make the movements of the galaxies pale in comparison. Moment-by-moment, millions of chemical reactions take place, each with a specific purpose, each working in harmony with others, each cell responding to feedback from the whole human organism. For the Christian, the study of physical life presents itself as a valid and powerful opportunity for worship, as God's intricacy and personality are so astoundingly reflected in the living things He has made.

Sometimes, however, the study of the body and the practice of medicine can be a frustrating and difficult journey for a physician. Human bodies have souls attached to them and when the body of someone you love is suffering, the objective work of a doctor becomes very, very personal. I understand this very well because ten years ago, a demanding medical "issue" infiltrated my very home, descending upon the body and soul of the one I care most about on this earth:

My wife Liz always thought that marrying a physician would improve her health. Who wouldn't like to have a personal doctor that does daily house calls? Boy, was she mistaken! For the first fifteen years of our marriage, Liz fought with a disease called "chronic fatigue/fibromyalgia." Year after year I watched as the illness slowly and persistently drained her energy and pulled her body into a continually exhausted state.

In the winter of 1995, she came down with very serious pneumonia. Even though the pneumonia eventually resolved, she was left with an overwhelming fatigue, as if the few remaining drops of energy in her body had evaporated. It left her completely drained of physical strength. She was unable to get out of bed for more than one or two hours a day.

She had also developed significant allergies and asthma. The only way she was able to go up to the barn and see her horses was to wear a large mask with double containers to filter the air. She looked like something out of the *War of the Worlds.* Mental fogginess distorted her ability to focus or concentrate on anything very long, making it difficult for her to read or even watch TV. So most of her days were filled with lying silently and simply allowing the time to pass.

Our three children took turns missing a day of school so they could care for her—much in the way that she had cared for them as babies. I tried everything I could think of. I studied, I researched, and I made phone calls. I took her to see four different medical specialists and they placed her on nine different prescription medications—yet the fatigue continued on month after month. When I would ask the specialists how long it would last, they would reply, "We just don't know. It could be several more months or it could be years. Ray, she may never get better." As a physician and a husband, I've never faced anything so difficult. I got frustrated, then I got apathetic; all I could do was stand by idly doing nothing, feeling helpless while she suffered. Even God did not seem to be hearing our prayers.

About this time a friend from a neighboring town visited Liz and shared with her that her husband had experienced severe fatigue following pneumonia several months earlier. He began taking nutritional supplements and his energy returned within months. She left some of the supplements with Liz and encouraged her to try them.

Liz, however, knew my personal feelings about supplements. For 23 years of my medical practice I had been telling my patients that if they would just eat the right kinds of food, they would not need any additional vitamins or supplements. After all, that's what I had been taught in medical school. (Actually, when I look back at my medical training, I was taught very little about nutrition and absolutely nothing about supplementation.) I regularly repeated the common phrase, "Vitamins just create expensive urine." You could spend a lot of money on them, but I felt they passed though the body with little effect. When Liz asked me about them, though, I was at the end. I said, "Honey, you can try anything you want. Nothing we doctors are doing is helping you."

She started the nutritional supplements and within a week she actually felt a *little* better. I was still skeptical, but the improvement continued. Within four or five weeks she was feeling much better and now off all of her medication. Within four to five months she was actually better than she had been in years. The husband in me was so thankful, but the doctor in me was so shocked. It was as if the Lord slapped me across the face and said, "Pay attention, Ray!" I was perplexed, not knowing whether her recovery was from a supernatural intervention of the Lord or if it could have been the result of nutrients and vitamins in the supplements she was taking. In any case, I was very humbled. When a physician is not able to help the one he loves the most, his pride takes a healthy beating.

The experience launched me into intense research regarding the health benefits of nutritional supplements. My findings and my application of this knowledge in my practice led to the writing of my first book, *What Your Doctor Doesn't Know about Nutritional Medicine* [Thomas Nelson 2002]. The book presents the medical evidence from hundreds of studies and tells the stories of the lives that are being touched when these findings are applied to their lives.

A Different World Now

When God walked and talked to Adam and Eve in the Garden of Eden, the world was much different. Prior to the invasion of sin and death, God described all He had made as "very good." So good that we see only broken fragments of it reflected today. Even the most magnificent displays of nature are nothing compared to the glory of His pure creation. So long ago and so far away...the perfection of what *was* is impossible for us to conceptualize through what *is* today. The soil was rich. The vegetation was lush. The air that they breathed was not polluted. Adam and Eve were at peace in their hearts and their minds, without shame or discord.

Today, one two-hour commute on the Santa Monica freeway will stand in sharp contrast to how it was in the beginning. Our stressful lives, polluted environment, depleted and highly processed diet, and overmedicated society have been attacking the very core of our health and our bodies. Satan desires to attack our bodies and our souls in an attempt to defeat our spirits. Whatever affects our physical bodies can also harm our souls, destabilizing the "temple" of the Holy Spirit. The vicious attack of free radicals on every cell in the body causes "oxidative stress" and inflammation—now known to be the root cause of over 70 chronic degenerative diseases. It's a problem that is amplified by any emotional stress or unresolved anger.

> Our stressful lives, polluted environment, depleted and highly processed diet, and overmedicated society have been attacking the very core of our health and our bodies.

"Resting in the Lord" and "setting the mind on the things above" reduces the oxidative stress caused by fear and worry. This decreases the excess free radical production in the body caused by emotional stress or unresolved anger. But we were never intended to live in a bubble. God has called us to a life of service and love...and that requires us to navigate through this toxic, stressful world. Because of stressful lifestyles, a polluted environment, and an overmedicated society, this generation must deal with more free radicals and oxidative stress than any previous generation that has walked the face of the earth.

Yet the body is not defenseless against this onslaught. God has designed us with a very complex "antioxidant" defense system, which counters the attack of free radicals, rendering them harmless. Some of these antioxidants are made by the body. Additional antioxidants are obtained from foods—primarily fruits and vegetables. After ten years of researching nutritional medicine, I'm convinced that the body's natural antioxidant defense system, natural immune system, and natural repair system are the best defense against developing chronic degenerative diseases. It is far more efficient and effective than any drugs I can prescribe.

God has called us to a life of service and love...and that requires us to navigate through this toxic, stressful world.

But the key question at this point is this: *Are we getting enough antioxidants from our food to prevent oxidative stress, or do we need nutritional supplements to accomplish this goal?* Overwhelmingly, the medical literature points to the fact that the human body's natural antioxidant system vitally needs the nutrients that supplements provide in order to do its job effectively. The absolute best way to optimize the natural defense systems is by supplementing the diet with high-quality, complete, and balanced nutritional supplements.

Essential nutrients are present in the foods of a healthy diet, but nutritional supplementation allows you to get them at levels you just can't get from foods today. *Nutritional supplementation allows you to optimize the healing power that God has already created and allows the body to function as God has designed.* This is what my wife Liz did and it allowed her to regain her health. My wife's healing was truly from the Lord. God has created the body with a tremendous ability to protect and heal itself, and the absolute best way to optimize the God-given natural defense systems is by eating a healthy diet, exercising consistently, resting in the Lord, and taking high-quality, complete, and balanced nutritional supplements.

This is in stark contrast to what I had learned in medical school and it is very different from what I told my patients for over 23 years. I now prescribe medication as a last resort and not a first choice. I now encourage my patients to begin eating a healthy diet and to develop a modest exercise program. I now encourage my Christian patients to learn to abide in Christ, rest in the Lord, and set their minds on the things above. And I now recommend that everyone who lives in this stressful, toxic world take high quality, complete, and balanced nutritional supplements—because we just can't get what the body needs from food anymore.

The Quality of Today's Food

Since the body manufactures antioxidants from the nutrients it gets from food and drinks, the quality and quantity of nutrients in food is of prime concern. It is a well-known fact that the quality of food has declined over the last few generations. Several reasons account for this:

Soil Depletion

Our soils are depleted in the nutrients they contain. They are especially low in essential mineral content. Rex Beach wrote this in his report to the United States Senate:

> "Do you know that most of us today are suffering from certain dangerous diet deficiencies, which cannot be remedied until the depleted soils from which we grow our foods are brought into proper mineral balance? The alarming fact is that foods—fruits and vegetables and grains—now being raised on millions of acres of land that no longer contain enough of certain minerals are starving us, no matter how much we eat."

Interestingly, Mr. Beach was addressing the seventy-fourth United States Congress in 1936! Since that time, we have done nothing to improve the situation; in fact, the situation is much worse. The majority of fertilizers used over the last 70 years are putting back only potassium, nitrogen, and phosphorous. This ignores the fact that the body requires five major minerals (calcium, magnesium, chloride, phosphorous, and potassium) and at least 16 trace minerals for optimal health. Plants cannot create minerals. They must absorb them from the soil. If our soils do not have the minerals, our plants will not have them either.

Due to economic issues, most farmers are more concerned about the volume of food they can produce rather than the nutrient content of the food and many are now producing more food of less value.

Preservation and Transportation

The food industry is able to provide a wide selection of fruits and vegetables throughout the year. The variety is good, the best on the planet. However, they are made available at a sacrifice. Most fruits and vegetables are "green harvested" before they are mature. The nutrients they would have absorbed on the tree or vine are lost as they ripen in the shipping crates. Shipping food over long distances also requires cold storage and other preservation methods, which further deplete the food of vital nutrients.

Processing and Preparation

The refinement process of our flour to create white bread or brown bread removes more than 23 essential nutrients from the wheat, magnesium being one of the most important. "Enriched" bread has about eight of these nutrients put back in, but the other 15 nutrients are never seen again. The fast food industry has jumped in and created great tasting food that is giving us mainly high-glycemic, high-fatty foods. Nearly 50 percent of the money we are spending on food today is fast food or convenience food. Typical fast foods are loaded with saturated fats, trans-fats, and high-glycemic carbohydrates. These foods not only lead to a carbohydrate addiction that can lead to obesity and diabetes but also they starve us to death nutritionally. French fries, soft drinks, and white bread buns contain very little in the way of vitamins, minerals, and antioxidants. Processed foods from the grocery store are not only high-glycemic but also significantly depleted of vital nutrients. Even store-bought whole foods lose much of their nutrients during preparation. Overcooking, dry storage, and freezing cause foods to lose nutritional value. Consider these facts:

1. Fresh salads and cut vegetables and fruits lose more than 40 to 50 percent of their value if they sit for more than three hours.
2. More than 80 percent of the magnesium in wheat is lost when the germ (outer portion of the grain) is removed in the process of making white flour.
3. Vitamin C is vulnerable to both heat and cold and is significantly depleted with prolonged storage.
4. Folic acid is significantly lost from food during the normal preparation.

Clearly, nutrients are in short supply in the foods we eat. The typical Western diet makes things even worse. In the last chapter, we discussed in detail what was involved in a healthy diet. Eating eight to 12 servings of fruits and vegetables, replacing the bad fat with the good fat, and avoiding high-glycemic and highly processed foods improves health *dramatically.* The medical literature shows that simply eating this amount of whole, fresh fruits and vegetables daily decreases the risk of heart disease, diabetes, cancer, stroke, Alzheimer's dementia, macular degeneration, and Parkinson's disease by *two to three fold!*

Unfortunately, most Americans do not eat or live this way. The Second National Health and Nutritional Survey (NHANES II) examined about 12,000 American adults and evaluated their eating habits. Here are some of their findings:

1. Seventeen percent of the population does not eat any vegetables.

2. Excluding potatoes and salads, 50 percent of the population does not eat any vegetables. In other words, only half of the population eats "garden" vegetables.
3. Only 41 percent have any fruit or fruit juices on a daily basis.
4. Only 10 percent of the population meets the USDA guidelines for eating a minimum of five servings of fruits and vegetables a day. (I recommend eight to 12 servings of fruits and vegetables.) Among African Americans, only 5 percent eat the recommended amount of fruits and vegetables.

Increased stress and pollution, depleted soil quality, and poor diets: These are all good arguments for the need to take nutritional supplements. But which ones do we need, and in what quantities?

RDA Versus Optimal or Advanced Levels of Nutritional Supplements

The Recommended Dietary Allowances (RDA) that you find on the labels of both food and vitamins were established in the late 1930s and 1940s as the *minimal* amounts of nutrients required to avoid an "acute deficiency disease." Acute deficiency diseases include scurvy (deficient in vitamin C), pellagra (deficient in niacin), and rickets (deficient in vitamin D). In the 1950s, the definition of RDAs was expanded to also include the minimal amount of nutrients required for normal growth and development.

The RDAs have done this job very well. The Centers for Disease Control no longer follows or reports the incidents of scurvy, pellagra, and rickets because the incidence of these diseases is now so low—most people don't even know what they are. *However, medical research is now showing us that the minimal levels of nutrients in the RDAs are ineffective in preventing chronic degenerative diseases.* For example, the RDA of vitamin E is 30 IU and yet you don't begin to see any health benefits in the medical literature until you begin supplementing at least 100 IU. These health benefits appear to continue to increase when supplementing your diet up to 400 IU of vitamin E .

So why don't you just go out and eat 400 IU of vitamin E from food? You would have to eat 33 pounds of spinach or 27 pounds of butter or 5 pounds of wheat germ each and every day, that's why! Similarly, vitamin C has an RDA of 60 mg, which is enough to prevent scurvy. However, measurable health benefits don't emerge in our medical literature until supplemental levels are increased to 1,000 to 2,000 mg daily. You would need to eat 16 medium oranges or 160 apples or 17 kiwi fruit to get that amount. (Bill and I both love kiwi fruit, but not that much!) Clearly, supplements are needed, even for those with a *healthy* diet. The need is amplified for those on the "normal" American diet. (The medical journal *Pediatrics* reported in September 1997 that only 1 percent of the children in the United States get the RDA levels of nutrients from their food!)

Yes, God created the body to live on certain micro- and macronutrients found in our foods. In Eden, everything that was required was available in abundance and oxidative stress was not an issue. In New York or New Deli, the only way to obtain these levels of nutrients our bodies require is to add nutritional supplements, even if we already have a healthy diet.

Cellular Nutrition

The goal of taking nutritional supplements is to have enough antioxidants in your system to neutralize the number of free radicals you produce. If you accomplish this goal, you are able to prevent oxidative stress, avoid inflammation, and go a long way in protecting your health from chronic degenerative disease.

Health Benefits of Nutritional Supplements

- Optimize your immune system
- Optimize your antioxidant defense system
- Optimize your natural repair system
- Decrease the risk of heart attacks and strokes
- Decrease the risk of cancer
- Decrease the risk of arthritis, macular degeneration, and cataracts
- Decrease the risk of asthma and hay fever
- Decrease the risk of Alzheimer's dementia, Parkinson's disease, and many other chronic degenerative diseases
- Improved sensitivity to your own insulin and help reverse insulin resistance and decrease the risk of developing diabetes

Providing the body with optimal or advanced levels of all nutrients is what I call "cellular nutrition." Cellular nutrition is defined as providing "optimal levels" (those levels that have been shown to provide a health benefit) of all these micronutrients to the cell. My basic nutritional supplementation recommendations are located in Table 1, which I believe provides this cellular nutrition.

TABLE 1		
Basic Nutritional Supplement Recommendations		
ANTIOXIDANTS	The more and varied your antioxidants, the better.	
VITAMIN A	I do not recommend the use of straight vitamin A because of its potential toxicity. I recommend supplementing with a mixture of mixed carotenoids. Carotenoids become vitamin A in the body as the body has need and they have no toxicity problems.	
CAROTENOIDS	It is important to have a nice mixture of carotenoids and not just to take beta-carotene.	
	• Beta-carotene	10,000 to 15,000 IU
	• Lycopene	1 to 3 mg
	• Lutein/Zeaxanthin	1 to 6 mg
	• Alpha carotene	500 mcg to 800 mcg
VITAMIN C	It is important to get a mixture of vitamin C, especially the calcium, potassium, zinc, and magnesium ascorbates, which are much more potent in handling oxidative stress.	
	• 1000 to 2000 mg	
VITAMIN E	It is important to be getting a mixture of vitamin Es. This should always be natural vitamin, and a mixture of natural vitamin is better: d-alpha tocopherol, d-gamma tocopherol, and mixed tocotrienol.	
	• 400 to 800 IU	
BIOFLAVANOID COMPLEX OF ANTIXODANTS	Bioflavanoids offer you a great variety of potent antioxidants. Having a variety of bioflavanoids is a great asset to your supplements. The amounts may vary but should include the majority of the following:	
	• Rutin	• Cruciferous
	• Quercitin	• Bilberry
	• Broccoli	• Grape-Seed Extract
	• Green Tea	• Bromelain
ALPHA-LIPOIC ACID	• 15 to 30 mg	
COQ10	• 20 to 30 mg	
GLUTATHIONE	• 10 to 20 mg	
	• Precursor: N-acetyl-L-cystein 50 to 75 mg	
B VITAMINS (COFACTORS)	• Folic Acid	800mcg
	• Vitamin B1 (Thiamin)	20 to 30 mg
	• Vitamin B2 (Riboflavin)	25 to 50 mg
	• Vitamin B3 (Niacin)	30 to 75 mg
	• Vitamin B5 (Pantothenic Acid)	80 to 200 mg
	• Vitamin B6 (Pyridoxine)	25 to 50 mg
	• Vitamin B12 (Cobalamin)	100mcg to 250mcg
	• Biotin	300mcg to 1,000mcg

TABLE 1
Basic Nutritional Supplement Recommendations

OTHER IMPORTANT VITAMINS	• Vitamin D3 (Cholecalciferol)	450 IU to 800 IU
	• Vitamin K 50 to 100 mcg	
MINERAL COMPLEX	• Calcium	800 to 1,500 mg (depending on your dietary intake of calcium)
	• Magnesium	500 mg to 800 mg
	• Zinc	20 to 30 mg
	• Selenium	200 mcg is ideal
	• Chromium	200 mcg to 300 mcg
	• Copper	1 to 3 mg
	• Manganese	3 to 6 mg
	• Vanadium	30 to 100 mcg
	• Iodine	100 mcg to 200 mcg
	• Molybdenum	50 mcg to 100 mcg
	• Mixture of Trace Minerals	
ADDITIONAL NUTRIENTS FOR BONE HEALTH	• Silicon	3 mg
	• Boron	2 to 3 mg
OTHER IMPORTANT AND ESSENTIAL NUTRIENTS Improved Homocysteine levels and improved brain function	• Choline	100 to 200 mg
	• Trimethylglycine	200 to 500 mg
	• Inositol	150 mg to 250 mg

SUPPLEMENTING YOUR DIET

ESSENTIAL FATS:	• Cold-Pressed Flaxseed oil	
	• Fish Oil Capsules	
FIBER SUPPLEMENT	• Blend of soluble and insoluble fiber	10 to 30 mg depending on your dietary comsumption fiber (ideal is 35 to 50 grams of total fiber daily)

**There are some nutritional companies who are putting together these essential nutrients into one or two different tablets, which need to be taken 2 to 3 times daily in order to achieve this level of supplementation. Look for a high-quality product that comes as close as possible to these recommendations. If the manufacturer follows pharmaceutical GMP and USP guidelines, you will be giving yourself the absolute best protection against oxidative stress.

The essential fats and fiber will give you the added nutrients that are usually missing in the Western diet.

Synergy

Cellular nutrition is a team effort where multiple nutrients work together for the greater cause utilizing a concept called "synergy," where the effectiveness of everything working together is much greater than the sum of their individual efforts. Synergy is the key to nutritional success. When you take in *all* the micronutrients the body needs at optimal levels, the nutrients are able to work more efficiently and their effectiveness increases dramatically. This again, is a reflection of the incredibly intricate and interconnected nature of all the systems of the body and the amazingly integrated chemistry that lies behind the scenes of physical life. When the antioxidants are used *together* and not alone (as they are in many of the clinical trials) one plus one does not equal two, but instead eight, 10, or even 20.

Supplementing with a balanced variety of 18 to 25 different antioxidants maximizes the effectiveness of each one. Different antioxidants work in different areas of the body and on different types of free radicals. There is no single "miracle" nutrient that does everything. They all work best together for the common good.

A study done at the University of Arizona supplemented the diet of a study group with 200 mcg of selenium and compared the results to a control group that did not receive selenium. The group that received the selenium decreased their risk of prostate cancer by 70 percent, decreased their risk of colon cancer by 60 percent, and lowered their risk of lung cancer by over 30 percent. As you might imagine, everyone ran out to buy selenium. People didn't realize, however, that the intracellular antioxidant, glutathione, was making the changes. Glutathione needs a molecule of selenium to work. You can have all the glutathione in the world in your cells, however, if you do not have enough selenium it cannot do its job as God intended. Remember, the goal is to have *all* the vital nutrients available to the cell at optimal levels.

Table 1 shows which nutrients are important and at what levels they should be taken. It's not necessary to go through costly or expensive testing to find out what you need a little more or a little less of. By choosing a nutritional supplement that is complete and balanced, and by taking it in sufficient amounts, you will provide the cells of your body with all the nutrients they need to function at their best possible level. Over time you will replenish nutritional deficiencies and bring all of the other nutrients up to their optimal levels so that the body can function as God designed it.

Some nutritional companies have combined all of the essential nutrients into one or two different tablets, which need to be taken two to three times a day. That saves a lot of calculating on your part. Check the labels and look for products that come as close as possible to the recommendations in Table 1.

Answers to Some Important Questions
Are nutritional supplements safe?

Every month, it seems, we hear a media report that challenges the effectiveness and safety of nutritional supplements—some even say that vitamin E or vitamin C is actually dangerous to your health! Researchers generally look at the effects of one or two nutrients during a study. (This is really the only way we can do research. If there are too many variables, it's impossible to tell which nutrient is causing which result.) The overwhelming majority of studies on a single nutrient show a statistically significant health benefit. However, there is a word of caution. When you use a particular nutrient alone at high doses, it can become a pro-oxidant, causing an increase in the number of free radicals produced. So occasionally we see a study that shows a negative result. (In my early years of medical practice, I would jump all over a negative study as proof of the dangers of taking vitamins and I would ignore the vast majority of studies that showed a health benefit.) As negative studies emerge, always note that they are done with either one or maybe two nutrients given at high doses. The broad consensus of the medical literature, however, shows that these reports do not apply to someone who is taking a balanced amount of all nutrients.

Nutritional supplements are safe. Complications from legal medication, on the other hand, cause over 180,000 deaths each and every year! (Tragically, over half of these deaths can and should be prevented if people just knew what to do.) For more information and detailed research regarding the dangers of medicine, read my book, *Death by Prescription* (Thomas Nelson 2003), available at www.drraystrand.com. Containing cutting edge research, this book explains how you can best prevent suffering or dying from an adverse drug reaction.

Cellular nutrition is a *critical* aspect of a healthy, proactive lifestyle. The bottom line is this: If you provide your body with *complete* and *balanced* supplements, you will see only health benefits.

How do I know I'm getting a good quality supplement?

The nutritional supplement industry is essentially unregulated. The Food and Drug Administration (FDA) monitors nutritional supplements as if they were a food. There is really no guarantee that what is on the label is actually in the pill. The government is definitely getting more serious about regulating the quality of nutritional supplements and the FDA is now looking into setting higher standards for the production of nutritional supplements—but it is going to take a few years to implement these new regulations. Until then, here are a few guidelines to help find the best available supplements from the most reliable companies:

Pharmaceutical-grade Good Manufacturing Practice (GMP)

Always select a company that manufactures their products using pharmaceutical-grade Good Manufacturing Practices. This means they purchase pharmaceutical-grade raw products and then manufacture them using pharmaceutical-grade standards. This is much the same way that drug companies produce over-the-counter drugs. Nutritional companies are not required to do this but some are now strictly following these guidelines. Pharmaceutical-grade GMP products give you the assurance that what's on the label is actually in the tablet. If companies follow only food-grade Good Manufacturing Practices, they need to have only 20 to 30 percent of what they say is on the label in the tablets. Don't get confused by their marketing strategies!

US Pharmacopoeia (USP).

It is also critical that tablets dissolve effectively. If they don't dissolve properly, the nutrients can't be digested and absorbed. (In that case, it really does not matter what is in them!) When nutritional companies follow USP guidelines, it gives you the assurance of the quality and potency of your supplements and that they are dissolving. Many nutritional companies do not follow USP guidelines. It's difficult to find out which products follow pharmaceutical-grade GMP and USP guidelines. You may need to look at their web site or even call the company directly and even then it is hard to get a straight answer. Companies that follow these guidelines are usually very proud of this fact and willing to share it readily. If you get a lot of double talk, they usually do not follow these guidelines. Nutritional companies that are international tend to have higher quality products as well.

Price is not always a good indicator of quality. Just because a supplement is high in price does not mean it is high in quality. But if you are serious about protecting your health, I would not sell yourself to the lowest bidder either. Look beyond hype, price, and marketing schemes. Find out about the company's adherence to GMP and USP guidelines and you will not go wrong.

Is nutritional supplementation "alternative medicine?"

The words "alternative medicine" conjure up all sorts of images. Cellular nutrition is not some anti-medical, on-the-fringe, dig-up-roots, chew-on-bat-wings mystical movement. The recommendations I am making are based on thousands of trials and studies reported in the most respected medical journals.

Nutritional supplementation isn't "medicine" either. It isn't prescribed to treat a particular disease. Supplements provide the cell what it needs to optimize your body's natural defense systems, allowing it to combat free radicals, lower oxidative stress, and help prevent chronic degenerative diseases. In that sense, it's not "alternative medicine," but it does prove to be complimentary medicine. Just as exercise and a healthy diet have significant health benefits, extensive medical research shows that high-quality, complete and balanced nutritional supplements offer great long-term health benefits when taken at optimal levels.

My findings, based on a decade of research and hundreds of medical studies, are recorded in my book, *What Your Doctor Doesn't Know about Nutritional Medicine,* (Thomas Nelson 2002). This work summarizes the findings of extensive medical trials and tests. It also explains why you are unlikely to hear about cellular nutrition from your physician!

Putting It All in Perspective

In the last three chapters, we've covered the three essential ingredients that allow us to optimize the bodies God has given us while on this earth: *exercise, healthy diet, and nutritional supplements.* As part of the overall plan for physical well being, nutritional supplements provide maximum health benefits when incorporated into a diet of good fats, good proteins, and good healthy, low-glycemic carbohydrates. Along with a consistent exercise program and learning to rest in the Lord, these healthy lifestyles give you the best opportunity to live life as God intended. That's the way He designed it, and any health benefits and health improvements you receive from living by this design can be seen as a gift of His grace and mercy. But let there be no doubt that this gift is given for a purpose far, far greater than our bodies themselves:

> *For we are His workmanship, created in Christ Jesus, for good works,*
> *which God prepared beforehand so that we would walk in them.*
> EPHESIANS 2:10

Far more important than the appearance or performance of our "earth suits" is the God who has brought us into a reconciled, forgiving relationship with Him.

As a tool of worship and an instrument of God's love working through you on earth, the body has certain earthly significance. Remember always, however, that your body is only a part of the equation—and it's the only *temporary* aspect of the spirit-soul-body design. Far more important than the appearance or performance of our "earth suits" is the God who has brought us into a reconciled, forgiving relationship with Him. That relationship in the Spirit is the ultimate gift, precious above all other things. It's the nucleus of all we have, all we have become, and all we are to do in this world and in the next, after this fallen body of flesh and bones is long forgotten.

PART FOUR

An Eternal Perspective

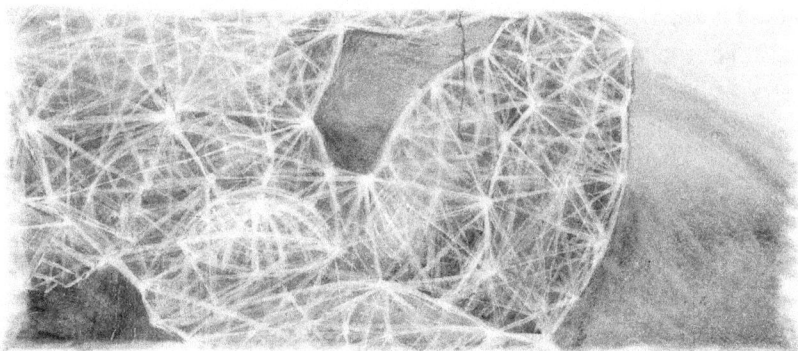

Yet you do not know what your life will be like tomorrow.

You are just a vapor that appears for a little while

and then vanishes away. Instead, you ought to say,

"If the Lord wills, we will live and also do this or that."

JAMES 4:14-15

The human body is a fabulous display of God's creativity and power—absolutely amazing when you look into its design and function. From the moment God formed humanity from the dust, and breathed His Spirit of life into our empty souls, we have represented the pinnacle of His creation and His affections. But let there be no doubt, these bodies were not given to us as ends in and of themselves. Your hands, your feet, your mind, and your tongue...your whole body is intended to be a tool of worship, an instrument of service, and a mouthpiece of love. The body you have is the only one you will ever get. In the last three chapters I gave you strong principles from the Bible and from medical science, exhorting you to care for it, discipline it, and feed it all that it needs, that your body might perform at its optimal capacity for all your days, be they many or few.

From here on, however, wisdom calls in a special way. Unless we live today in light of the future, our days will drift past in a meaningless fog, our trials and struggles will be misinterpreted, and the end of this earthly existence will be a struggle and a fight to keep something that was never ours in the first place. The spirit-soul-body design takes on new meaning as we look to the future. The future of the human body is destined for pain, illness, and death. For the spirit, the future holds perfection, power, and eternal life and the expectations we take with us into this future will determine the level of peace and vision of our souls today.

Eternal God and Father,

As we turn now to the uncertainty of the future, we ask that You would speak to us from Your Word through Your Spirit. Teach us about Your plan in this fallen world. Give us principles to live day to day. Show us our hopes that are based on lies and false expectations; that we might reject them. Teach us of the hope that has been determined by Your will from all eternity; that we might embrace it.

We pray that the eyes of our hearts might be enlightened, that we might know what is the hope of Your calling, what are the riches of the glory of Your inheritance in the saints, and what is the surpassing greatness of Your power toward us who believe (Ephesians 1:18-19).

Amen.

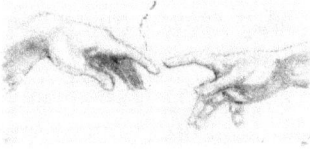

CHAPTER 10

Healing God's Way

Is anyone among you suffering? Let him pray. Is anyone cheerful?

Let him sing praises. Is anyone among you sick? Let him call for

the elders of the church, and let them pray over him, anointing him

with oil in the name of the Lord; and the prayer offered in faith will

restore the one who is sick, and the Lord will raise him up,

and if he has committed sins, they will be forgiven him.

JAMES 5:13-15

In the world you have tribulation.

JESUS CHRIST, JOHN 16:33

Somewhere in the course of our Christian journey, most of us have picked up the idea that life on earth is supposed to be easy, secure, and pleasant. Some television preachers proclaim the Christian life can (and should) be free from struggles, pain, difficulty, and loss. Books promise victory in seven simple steps. Honestly, don't you wish for a life where miracles happen continually and our problems are solved overnight? (Personally, I think miracles do happen continually, just not every time we want one, or not necessarily in the way we want them.)

Now that we are "saved" and God is "on our team," we would like to believe that we've been elevated to some sort of insulated earthly plane, a place where the Spirit protects and God provides just like we've always hoped someone would. We've always yearned for someone who anticipates our every desire, who stands by moment-by-moment to make sure that all our preferences became realities. Isn't God supposed to be that someone? Yet on Sunday mornings we put on our best smile and try to conceal our disappointment, because God isn't coming through for us the way we want.

Life, it turns out, is filled with trials, tribulation, and illness. Where we long for stability, we find chaos and upheaval. When we long for excitement, repetitive monotony descends. We are surprised by pain, as if our faith should shield us from difficulty before it can get to us. When we aren't living a prosperous, easy life, we feel that we must be doing something wrong. Perhaps we lack faith? Are we missing the formula that will persuade God to release a flow of blessings and resources that fulfill our dreams?

Society itself has laid out a similar expectation: If we do our part, work hard, invest in the right stocks, and are covered by the right insurance, then we will be protected from hardship and loss. In the end, we spend tremendous amounts of energy and passion fighting for something that we will never have, and were never designed to know: a life without difficulty. Even if you follow a healthy diet, exercise, take nutritional supplements, and abide in Christ, this "earth suit" will someday become ill and eventually die.

When You Become Ill

I have been involved in a private family practice for over 31 years. It's the nature of my work to deal with those who are ill. Many of my patients have been strong Christians and I have been involved with them personally in their pain and suffering. Face to face, as we walk together through both healing and death, I've been able to witness how believers approach their illnesses. I have seen those who place their entire hope in doctors and modern medicine. I have also seen those who totally ignore my advice and turn to unusual alternative medical care. I have also seen those with tremendous faith who choose not submit to any traditional medical treatment, but instead completely rely on their faith alone.

In the midst of it all, I have learned not to pass judgment. Illness strikes at the very core of our physical existence. Those who face it often do so in desperation (and sometimes in denial), but they always seek to make the

best decisions they can in good conscience...and they often do so in compli-
cated circumstances.

Watching others walk through illness has given me plenty of motivation
to search the Scriptures, seeking how God would want me to approach my
own personal illness, when it comes. God's Word is living and active, and has
much to say when it comes to tribulations, trials, and illness. Key principles
from the Bible offer firm, yet general, guidelines to all who are (or will) face
illness and disease.

Is anyone among you sick? Let him call for the elders of the church,
and let them pray over him, anointing him with oil in the
name of the Lord; and the prayer offered in faith will restore
the one who is sick, and the Lord will raise him up,
and if he has committed sins, they will be forgiven him.
JAMES 5:14-15

From this passage, we can draw three guidelines to follow when facing
an illness.

1. Accept It

According to Spiros Zodhiates, Th.D, James 5:14 begins by making an
assumption. "Is anyone among you sick?" It is as much of a statement as it
is a question, pointing to the universal fact that people get sick. While many
of us would like to believe that illness is not the norm, the Bible says differently. Even the apostle Paul struggled with an ongoing disability, even though
he wrote about the gift of healing in 1 Corinthians and was an instrument
through whom God healed many. Barring an early "accidental" death, illness
should be expected by all of us. It's not a matter of *if,* only a matter of
when...and the Christian is not exempt. When 2 Corinthians 4:16 states that
the "outer man is decaying," it means just that. The body is wearing away
like a piece of tattered clothing (Isaiah 51:6). And unless we live to see the
rapture (which is a real possibility), illness will one day bring us to the point
of death.

And inasmuch as it is appointed for men
to die once and after this comes judgment.
HEBREWS 9:27

Think about the many people who received miraculous physical healing at the hand of Christ during His three years of ministry. Where are their mortal bodies today? Are they still living? What about Lazarus, whom Christ raised from the dead? Is Lazarus still alive? Obviously, the answer is "no." They have all shared in the same physical death you and I will share (unless the Lord returns soon). In order to have a proper perspective of the future and realistic expectations for the present, it is important to remember that our physical bodies will die some day.

2. Seek Competent Medical Help

At the time of the apostolic church, the elders performed many duties, including treating the sick. According to the original Greek, Dr. Zodhiates' interprets James 5:14 in this way:

> What are these elders to do when they come to a home of a
> sick brother? "Let them pray on him or over him." But before
> they pray, they must render whatever medical or physical
> therapeutic assistance they can. The order to the two things
> that the elders are supposed to do is not made clear from the
> [English] translation, but it is absolutely clear from the Greek
> text. The word translated "anointing him" is in the aorist
> participle, aleipsantes, which makes it an act which precedes
> the prayer, "having rubbed him with oil." Oil in the Scriptures is
> used for religious anointing as well for lighting and medicinal
> purposes. In this situation, the word "chrio" is used. This
> means to rub or apply ointment. Therefore, this refers to the
> application of medicinal assistance first to the sick person,
> and then the elders are commanded to pray for the sick.

According to the James passage, then, the sick are to seek medical advice and treatment as they are initiating a call to the elders of the church. Some Christians wonder if the Bible prohibits the use of medication or medical treatments. I can find no verses to support this, and I personally believe that there should be no hesitation in seeking medical advice or treatment when you become ill. The person you consult may not be a medical doctor. Advice could be from a naturopath, chiropractor, or even some other alternative health care provider. Even though I am a medical doctor, I do not feel that physicians have a monopoly on medical knowledge and treatment. I have seen many patients whose health is significantly improved by alternative or non-mainstream therapy. That being said, I have also seen many patients find significant improvement in their health and suffering through traditional medical care. Whatever your choice, you should seek competent medical care and advice.

3. Pray in the Name of the Lord

Zodhiates goes on to state that there is a restrictive qualification as to the possible result of the application of medicine and the offering of prayer in regard to a believing, sick person for our prayers are to be "in the name of the Lord" (5:14):

> The phrase "in the name of the Lord" does not refer to a matter of habit by which one must close his prayers. It indicates a willingness to place prayer under the sovereign will and purpose of God. His best may include sickness and privation instead of health and wealth, but it is designed to bring the believer into a closer walk with Him.

Jesus modeled this powerful principle to us in the lonely hours before His brutal death, when He prayed, "My Father, if it is possible, let this cup pass from Me; yet not as I will, but as You will" (Matthew 26:39). In John 14:13 our Lord said, "And whatever you ask in My name, that will I do, so that the Father may be glorified in the Son." Luke 11:9 calls us to, "Ask, and it will be given to you." The word "ask" in this verse is the same Greek word from which we derive the verb "to beg." We are to come to the Lord as a beggar would to a generous giver. We cannot demand, but only make our needs known to God and God will give to us according to His will and discernment. The Lord certainly gives us the freedom and commands us to pray for all that we wish our heavenly Father should do for us. But our heavenly Father, knowing more and better than we do, does not necessarily give us the health and wealth we ask for, but that which He knows is the best for us.

It is a matter of faith and trust. Once we have been obedient to follow His word and direction by seeking medical help and anointing our situation with prayer, the results are to be left up to God. He is a prayer-hearing and prayer-answering God, yet this verse does not give us a blanket authorization to demand anything from God. We can pray and ask God to intervene supernaturally. And we must pray and ask in full dependence upon God's perfect

He will give us only what is for our eternal good. But what is good for the believer in God's eyes may not be what the believer desires.

awareness of our real needs, trusting that He will act according to His wisdom.

He will give us only what is for our eternal good. But what is good for the believer in God's eyes may not be what the believer desires. In light of this, our faith and trust in God must be based on the fact that His plans for us are good and not evil. While Romans 8:28 has almost become a worn-out cliché, its promise still gives hope to those who claim its truth and apply its promise to situations in which we can see no earthly good:

> And we know that God causes all things to work together
> for good to those who love God,
> to those who are called according to His purpose.

His purpose is that we might know Him and be conformed to the likeness of His dear Son, and often it is illness and suffering itself that accomplishes this very thing.

It is God who heals all people, unbelievers and believers alike, with or without medicine. In the case of the believer, however, there must be the realization that after the application of medicine and then prayer, we must release the results to Him. God is sovereign, and we are to place our hurt and suffering in His hands knowing that He is also good, and will work our situation to His glory.

God Can and Does Heal

My Uncle Albert was a tough, hearty man who had been seasoned by years as a farmer on the Dakota plains. At the age of 62, however, it looked as though physical life was over for him. He was diagnosed with advanced prostate cancer. Doctors tried to radiate it, but when nothing helped, they told him that he had less than six months to live. They said that it was time to go home and get his affairs in order, that there was nothing left to do.

But Albert knew that there was something left to do. He gathered with the elders from his home church in the huge metropolis of Platte, South Dakota (population at that time a whopping 1,500, if you counted cats and dogs). They laid hands on Albert and asked God if He wouldn't heal him. God intervened and granted the desire. Uncle Albert went on to live a full life; God granting him an additional 24 years. He was a strong man of faith and many lives were touched by his sweet spirit and love.

I admitted my Uncle Albert into the hospital at the age of 86 for pneumonia. When I did his admission physical, the prostate tumor was still there, still rock hard, but it hadn't advanced at all! I'd never seen anything like it. In fact, I walked out of his hospital room and ran into our local urologist. I asked him to examine Albert. The urologist could not find any advanced spread even though his prostate was the worst feeling prostate he had ever examined.

Albert did eventually die the following year because of the prostate cancer, but in response to his request, God had granted him more than two extra decades of life.

When God Says "No"

Arouse Yourself, why do You sleep, O Lord?
Awake, do not reject us forever. Why do You hide
Your face and forget our affliction and oppression?
PSALM 44:23-24

So, let's say you've gotten sick. According to James, you "accept" the reality of the illness, seek competent medical intervention, and pray for healing...and yet the illness persists. Where do you go from there? Tim Hansel, in his book, *You Gotta Keep Dancing,* describes the reality of unanswered prayer, broken dreams, and challenging circumstances in vibrant colors. He knows them well. A mountain climbing accident has made intense back pain his constant companion. He also knows the tearing, searing agony of broken relationships and difficult marriage struggles:

Pain. We all know what it tastes like. Whether its
source is physical, emotional, mental, or spiritual, its inter-
ruption in our lives disrupts and reshapes. It intercepts our
hopes and plans; it rearranges our dreams. It always leaves a
mark. I realize again each day that all of our physical lives
are terminal. Only time and quality differ. The choice for all
of us is not if we will accept pain, but how.

The first state is denial—not believing that it's really
happening. The second state is bargaining, trying to equivo-
cate with God to make deals. The third stage is anger, the

rage that comes from within based upon frustration, which
cannot be satiated. The fourth stage is depression, a symp-
tom of both prolonged anger turned inward and guilt. The
final stage is acceptance, realizing that what is, IS—and is
going to be.

The Bible, in particular, makes no claim that life in this world is going to be easy and smooth. Quite to the contrary, difficulty is assumed to be the normal mode of operation. Unwanted health problems, depression from the loss of something or someone we deeply desired, the heaviness of spiritual warfare...all are the norm in Scripture. But thankfully, God doesn't leave us floundering, searching for our own devices of deliverance. The Bible is full of practical principles and specific advice for those who are willing to accept tribulation as part of the equation of life, and respond to it as God designed.

Perhaps more than anything else, suffering exposes our true inner beliefs about God and our actual expectations about life. When times get tough, all our thoughts and hopes for fairness, fullness, and comfort on earth come to the surface. In the midst of the difficulty our desires scream out for help and healing from a God that we believe and know can do anything.

As believers, we know that we do not always get from God all that we ask. We know that if it was God's purpose and timetable to allow this physical body to live forever in health, He could do it. We know that our bodies are vulnerable to illness and will succumb to death. We know all that, but still, when God doesn't do what we want, our hearts are often filled with great disappointment. Certainly there are times when God doesn't "fix" our problems or meet our needs as we wish He would. Relationships remain broken and bills go unpaid. Even after eating right and exercising appropriately still we may not look the way we want. Even after prayer and medical attention, our bodies often continue to suffer illness.

While we wish that God would heal and deliver every time, He often chooses not to. His choice to not heal seems to have little to do with our level of faith in Him. Paul, on at least one occasion, was delayed in his travels because of sickness, and in 2 Corinthians mentioned a "thorn in the flesh, a messenger of Satan to buffet me...I implored the Lord three times that it might leave me" (2 Corinthians12:7-8).

God's choices even appear to have little to do with our level of devotion and godliness. The Old Testament prophet Asaph was very frustrated by

God's apparent unfairness in this matter. He said, "I was envious of the arro-
gant as I saw the prosperity of the wicked. For there are no pains in their
death...They are not in trouble as other men, nor are they plagued like
mankind" (Psalm 73:3-5). Solomon shared this observation in Ecclesiastes
7:14-15:

*In the day of prosperity be happy, but in the day
of adversity consider-God has made the one as well as the other...
I have seen everything during my lifetime of futility;
there is a righteous man who perishes in his righteousness
and there is a wicked man who prolongs his life in his wickedness.*

I wish I could offer you a fail-safe formula (complete with a money-back
guarantee) that would give you a healthy, struggle-free life on this planet. But
quite frankly, the formula just doesn't exist. Ultimately, God is the One that
holds our lives in His hands. For reasons that we may never understand on
this side of heaven, He is often the healer who chooses not to heal, the
provider who withholds, and the deliverer that allows us to remain in the battles. He never promised differently, and examples from the Word and from
the evening news illustrate what we already know: Life will dish out all the
pain and suffering it can muster. It's not a matter of if, but only when it will
come.

The healing that my wife Liz experienced as the result of taking nutritional supplements astounded both of us. But just recently, she suffered a
stroke. We thank God that she has recovered well, but as she and I age, illness and injury seem to be coming at us with greater frequency and intensity.

Twenty years ago, Bill's brother Dick was wrestling with severe depression. Dick was the first Christian on that side of the family, and God worked
through him to reach hundreds, if not thousands of people for Christ. But
when the darkness set in, it was fierce. Bill remembers it this way:

*Dick put himself in a hospital where he was under
constant care and observation. Dozens of us were intensely
praying for him and for his healing and he seemed to be on
the edge of a breakthrough. But one day, a doctor left him
with a full bottle of potent antidepressants. That night, Dick
made plans for his own funeral, wrote a letter declaring the
goodness of God, and penned his farewell to us. He then
swallowed all the pills.*

That was over two decades ago and the pain of his loss
still burns in our friends' and family's hearts. I have no
expectation that it will fully go away until we are with him
again in heaven.

If you do everything we suggest in this book, I believe you will be the better for it. I have seen hundreds of my Christian patients literally regain their health by "living by design." However, you will not be insulated from the absolute certainty of trials, broken dreams, and disappointed hope. Actually, that is clearly part of the design.

Jesus promises that in this world "you will have tribulation"—but that's not His only promise. The promise of suffering is wrapped in words of hope and power that are at the core of God's design. As we align ourselves to this design, something truly supernatural emerges from the ashes.

These things I have spoken to you, so that in Me
you may have peace. In the world you have tribulation,
but take courage; I have overcome the world.
JOHN 16:33

Jesus has a way with words, doesn't He! Only God's Son could get away with a message like that. Who else could tell us, "Relax; life is difficult; get used to it." But then, only God's Son has been here and back. He alone has felt the crushing weight of the world's sin—and only He has transformed the drops of blood into a river of forgiveness. He alone has felt the darkness and isolation of death—and only He has returned to prove and proclaim that He has transcended it.

Yes, Jesus alone could promise us pain and struggle—and then tell us to embrace it with His peace and with courage. Could it be that this Jesus is breaking through our superficial and temporary longings for a comfortable and easy life in order to bring us into something that is spiritually real, eternal, and impenetrable?

Paul thought so. Though his three pleas for deliverance from his circumstances went unanswered, he knew that something infinitely more important was being given:

Concerning this, I implored the Lord three times
that it might leave me. And He has said to me,
"My grace is sufficient for you, for power is perfected in weakness."
Most gladly, therefore, I will rather boast about my weaknesses,
so that the power of Christ may dwell in me.
Therefore I am well content with weaknesses, with insults,
with distresses, with persecutions, with difficulties,
for Christ's sake; for when I am weak, then I am strong.
2 CORINTHIANS 12:8-10

Somehow, in a way that makes little worldly sense, Jesus uses hardship to invite us into a dance with Him that has absolutely no earthly equal. The invitation calls us to stand up, get off the chair of circumstances, and free ourselves from our desires to have our circumstances changed. He invites us to join Him on the stage in a ballet that changes us through our circumstances as He lifts us above our struggles. As pain draws us closer to His side, He leads this new dance, showing us new steps to new music, where in our weakness He is shown strong as the power of Christ permeates our being.

Perhaps it is the greatest image we can offer the world of the inner reality of God in our souls. In adversity we vacate our dreams, allow the Spirit to occupy our thoughts, align our will to God's, then choose to allow Jesus to live it out through our pain in His power.

But not only does it communicate the reality of God to those around us, the dance also frees us to experience life in new ways. Tim Hansel, described the transition this way in *Gotta Keep Dancing:*

Slowly my rage to live emerged from the depression,
frustration, and anger. But when it was there I realized that
it had a taste to it that I'd never known before. I began to
see life in a way that never would have been possible before.
I began to relish small, daily, simple things, and realized at a
depth that never seemed possible that all of life was sacred.
There were moments, though sporadic and far apart, when I
began to understand that life wasn't over for me, but perhaps
was just beginning.

Time and time again, we have heard stories about how embracing both pain and Christ unleashes a vivid and focused vision for moment-by-moment joy and wonder. The struggle forces us to become better rather than bitter, to gaze at God rather than fixate on our condition. The certainty of tribulation in this life may be one of the great realizations that allow us to quit fighting for things that never will be and jump in feet first into the here and now, cherishing every second of the day.

> **The certainty of tribulation in this life may be one of the great realizations that allow us to quit fighting for things that never will be and jump in feet first into the here and now, cherishing every second of the day.**

One of my wife's and my dearest friends is Peggy Wipf. She's always exercised, watched her eating, and has a heart for the things of God. At the age of 38 however, Peggy's body descended into a series of illnesses that has lasted for nearly 16 years now. She developed insulin dependent diabetes and quickly suffered complications that have affected the nerves to her bowels and legs. This has caused her bowels to pretty much stop working and has left her legs in continual pain. There have been healings along the way. Some appeared to be miraculous and many came through the caring hands of doctors. As we write this book, Peggy has faced kidney failure due to her diabetes and has recently had a kidney and pancreas transplant. She continues to be very weak and suffers greatly.

Through all her struggles, she has found the ability to dance in Christ. Though her flesh falters and fails her, her heart continually finds strength and joy in God's promises and presence (Psalm 73:26). Remarkably, there is not only enough joy for her, but enough to overflow from her toward those of us fortunate enough to know her.

Some time ago, she sent me a list of verses that pull her through each day, even as she longs to be physically free and to be at home with the Lord. Here are three of our favorites:

> *The cords of death encompassed me,*
> *And the torrents of ungodliness terrified me.*
> *The cords of Sheol surrounded me; The snares of death confronted me.*
>
> *In my distress I called upon the LORD,*
> *And cried to my God for help; He heard my voice out of His temple,*
> *And my cry for help before Him came into His ears.*
>
> PSALM 18:4-6

Behold, the eye of the LORD is on those who fear Him,
On those who hope for His lovingkindness,
To deliver their soul from death,
And to keep them alive in famine.
Our soul waits for the LORD;
He is our help and our shield.
For our heart rejoices in Him,
Because we trust in His holy name.
Let Thy lovingkindness, O LORD, be upon us,
According as we have hoped in Thee.

PSALMS 33:18-22

Who will protect me from the wicked? Who will stand up
for me against evildoers? Unless the LORD had helped me,
I would soon have died. I cried out, "I'm slipping!"
and your unfailing love, O LORD, supported me. When doubts
filled my mind, your comfort gave me renewed hope and cheer.

PSALM 94:16-19

Passages such as these promise the things that we look for in good circumstances. Isn't it interesting that the Word says that perhaps they can be found only in *difficult* ones? This is the real stuff, not some sort of consolation prize for losers. God doesn't give difficulty reluctantly, and we are not to accept it grudgingly. Through struggles we find the peace, the purpose, the power, and the focus that we've been looking for.

In time, we will be able to look back and see clearly God's goodness in the midst of the hurt. But for now, it requires faith. Joseph had been given promises of great power and position in a dream from God (Genesis 37). Yet for the next three chapters, his life was full of graphic betrayal by brothers, abandonment into slavery, and imprisonment on false charges. But Joseph held strong to the promises and lived to see God's purpose in his journey. In the end he was a blessing to his enemies and was able to comfort them with these words:

Do not be afraid, for am I in God's place? As for you,
you meant evil against me, but God meant it for good in order
to bring about this present result, to preserve many people alive.

GENESIS 50:19-20

Joseph lived to see what he held to only by faith during the dark days. For some of our trials, we may need to look back from the perspective of eternity to see the redemption of our personal history. Yet in the here and now, we can choose His joy and know His peace that transcends our struggles. When we live by His design, we can do more than survive; we can thrive in the midst of hardship, embracing difficulties as an instrument of His love. In spite of the worst of circumstances, we are always better off as we walk through them with a clear awareness of His presence and His holy sovereignty.

Good emerging from evil. Beauty radiating from scars. Power flowing out of weakness. These are the wonders and the realities for those who choose to dance with Christ in the midst of difficulty and broken dreams.

Good emerging from evil. Beauty radiating from scars. Power flowing out of weakness. These are the wonders and the realities for those who choose to dance with Christ in the midst of difficulty and broken dreams.

God has given us many tools to use against the struggles that we face. The effective prayer of a righteous person "can accomplish much" (James 5:16), as can the wise words of a trustworthy counselor. The skilled hand of a doctor and the advancements of modern medicine offer hope as well. Healthy eating, proper exercise, nutritional supplementation, and forgiveness are all wise choices that can eliminate many unnecessary and unwanted afflictions. God will continue to intervene supernaturally and miraculously heal many who are suffering illness and pain.

But let there be no mistake, difficult times will be ours until the last of our breath has passed over our lips. Between now and then, may the glory and the wonder of God be yours, may His goodness permeate your pain, and may His hope dominate your wishes.

Before the winds that blow do cease, teach me to dwell within Thy calm:
Before the pain has passed in peace, give me, my God, to sing a psalm.
Let me not lose the chance to prove, the fullness of enabling love.
O Love of God, do this for me:
Maintain a constant victory.
Before I leave the desert land, for meadows of immortal flowers,
Lead me where streams at Thy command, flow by the borders of the hours.
That when the thirsty come, I may show them the fountains in the way.
O Love of God, do this for me:
Maintain a constant victory.

AMY CARMICHAEL

Make me to hear joy and gladness,
let the bones which You have broken rejoice.

PSALM 51:8

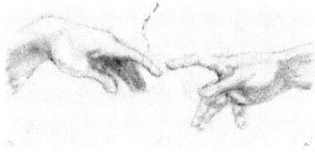

CHAPTER 11

Eternal Eyes

"...we look not at the things which are seen, but at the things

which are not seen; for the things which are seen are temporal,

but the things which are not seen are eternal."

2 CORINTHIANS 4:18

In the beginning, God created. All we see, all we feel, all we sense...everything that exists found its genesis in the heart of the infinite, eternal, all-knowing, and all-powerful One we call God. The heavens above, the earth below, the trees, the clouds, the roaring of the rivers, the animals...all is of His making. As the pinnacle of His work and in the image of Himself, God created humanity. With a spirit, soul, and a body He fashioned us, designing us for intimacy with Him. Our first ancestors walked with Him for a season in the perfection of all He had made. Now, through the rebellion of Adam and Eve so long ago and the continual sin of our flesh today, we live far, far away from the purity of Eden. Stuck as we are between the perfection of the garden and the promise of heaven, our existence on this earth is one of stress, decay, and eventually physical death.

In the preceding pages Bill and I have shared key principles for "living by design." We have drawn these principles from God's holy, unchanging Word and from the ever advancing and changing world of medical science. We believe that what we have shared can enable each of us to regain and experience much of God's original plan, even in the midst of this decaying and dying world. Our sincere prayer is that these words will bring health, life, and freedom in substantial measure. Our hope is this: that you be delivered from the bondage of anger by forgiveness; that you will find yourself free from the trap of self-effort; that you will find true rest in the Lord; and that your heart will find peace and vision as you set your mind on the things above. Our desire is that through exercise, a healthy diet, and nutritional supplements, your body will be an effective tool in God's hand as you allow Him to use it to worship, serve, and love.

> *...life makes sense only when we begin to see beyond what we can see. In order to live by design, we must look with "eternal eyes."*

But please, please know that that is not the end of it. *Our health and our peace on this earth were never designed to be an end in and of themselves.* We were created for something beyond this earthly existence, and our true design finds true meaning only when we look at life in the here-and-now through eternal eyes. In fact, *life makes sense only when we begin to see beyond what we can see.*

In order to live by design, we must look with "eternal eyes."

The Creation of Time

As I write this chapter, I am turning 60 years old. My friend and coauthor, Bill, is now 52 years old. I don't *feel* that old and find it hard to believe that the decades have passed me by so quickly. I am not over-the-hill-yet. However, I am certainly "on the back nine" (a term golfers will understand!). Where did the years go?! When I was young, I remember thinking 40 was *really* old. Now as I look toward the 70s and 80s, 40 seems so, so far behind me. Certainly, age teaches each of us the same lesson: Time passes quickly and waits for no man or woman.

Here on earth we are time creatures (time being one of the greatest creations of God). It is the great equalizer. No matter what your position is here on this earth—regardless of your wealth, your power, your influence, or lack of these things—you have only so much time. And Scripture is very clear that this time is fleeting.

As for man, his days are like grass; as a flower of the field,
so he flourishes. When the wind has passed over it,
it is no more, and its place acknowledges it no longer.
PSALM 103:15-16

God alone knows how much time we have to live here on this earth. He knows the number of our days before we are even born. What else would you expect from an all-powerful and all-knowing God?

Thine eyes have seen my unformed substance;
and in Thy book they were all written, the days that were
ordained for me, when as yet there was not one of them.
PSALM 139:16

God only knows how the end will come for you. Perhaps it will be in a hospital. Perhaps it will happen today at a busy intersection during rush hour traffic. Perhaps we will be the generation that lives to see the return of Christ. Though the circumstances are unknown, one truth is unavoidable. Life as we know it will not last.

While diet, exercise, and supplements can improve the quality of our lives here on earth, nothing will divert us from death's certain grip. God's supernatural healing may allow us to temporarily avert death, but He has chosen to allow all of us to face it, barring the rapture. According to Proverbs 3:1-2, wisdom will add length of days and years to your life, And peace they will add to you. However, the end of this existence will come. Moses confessed that, "As for the days of our life, they contain seventy years, or if due to strength, eighty years...For soon it is gone and we fly away" (Psalm 90:10).

In order to fully live by design, it is important that physical death is seen as one of the universal and unavoidable facts of life. When our beliefs and our hearts become aligned with truth, freedom results every time. John wrote that, "You shall know the truth, and the truth shall make you free" (John 8:32). But let's be honest; most of us are in bondage to the fear of death. We divert ourselves from its reality, and we deny its inevitability. We may even intentionally fill our lives with noise and activity to numb ourselves from its certainty. We cling to our earthly existence as if it is the only thing we have...and the stress this causes is incredible, potentially accelerating the aging process we are trying to avoid. Many a good day is fretted away in worry as we try to protect something that was never ours, as we fight to pre-serve something that will never last.

And which of you by being anxious can add
a single cubit to his life's span?
MATTHEW 6:27

Freedom from this fear is a central and logical conclusion in light of the Gospel. Christ came to earth for this very reason:

...that through death He [Christ] might render powerless
him who had the power of death, that is, the devil,
and might free those who through the fear
of death were subject to slavery all their lives.
HEBREWS 2:14-15

Because of what Christ accomplished on the Cross, we need not approach the grave with avoidance or fear. We can face our earthly end with focus and anticipation.

Because of what Christ accomplished on the Cross, we need not approach the grave with avoidance or fear. We can face our earthly end with focus and anticipation. At death, the union the body has with the soul and spirit is broken. Finally separated from the failing body of flesh, the soul and spirit are set free for eternity and they are set free in ways that we can't even imagine. At this point the "design of life" completely changes for the Christian. As we leave time behind and enter eternity, incalculable realities become the new norm. Those realities will be experienced then, but they can and should alter the way we perceive and experi-ence life on this side of the grave.

Promises for Over the Horizon

I was 33 years of age when I committed my life to the Lord. After my spir-itual birth there were many changes in my life. One of the more drastic was my change in attitude and perception toward physical death. No longer was death a desperate end to life and an entrance into nothingness. Instead I began to see it as a beautiful transition...one that is necessary to truly be at home and pres-ent with the Lord in fullest measure. To the Christian, death does not (and should not) have the same hold that it does for the nonbeliever. Because of

Christ's sacrifice on the Cross, the believer now has victory over sin and victory over death. In that single breathtaking truth we find hope—not only for the future, but also for today. Paul put it in perspective with these words:

> *Therefore, being always of good courage, and knowing*
> *that while we are at home in the body we are absent from*
> *the Lord—for we walk by faith, not by sight—we are of good courage,*
> *I say, and prefer rather to be absent from the body*
> *and to be at home with the Lord.*
> 2 CORINTHIANS 5:6-8

> *'O death, where is your victory? O death, where is your sting?'...*
> *but thanks be to God, who gives us the victory*
> *through our Lord Jesus Christ.*
> 1 CORINTHIANS 15:55, 57

Death itself was defeated by Christ on the Cross! In Him we have triumph over our most feared enemy. He conquered sin and the grave by the cleansing sacrifice of His blood. He proved that He had done so when He left behind an empty tomb. Jesus proclaimed, "I am the resurrection and the life; he who believes in Me will live even if he dies, and everyone who believes in Me will never die" (John 11:25-26).

> It's one of the most amazing aspects of Christianity, one that separates it from all other religions of the world: We worship a living Lord.

It's one of the most amazing aspects of Christianity, one that separates it from all other religions of the world: We worship a *living* Lord. Jesus is not a dead prophet. Jesus is alive. He has risen from the grave. He is the beginning, the firstborn from the dead (Colossians 1:18). While we might stumble and falter in the sinfulness of our flesh, and while our bodies will undergo certain decay and illness, Christians can boldly face death knowing that victory was made complete on the Cross. We can shout "Halleluiah!!" We can shout, "O death, where is your victory? O death, where is your sting?" For those who have made the decision to accept Christ as their Savior, physical death is not the end; it's only the beginning.

When All Is Made New, Again

In Scripture, a new beginning is unveiled in the last two chapters of

Revelation—and what an unveiling it is! We catch a glimmer of "a new heaven and a new earth" (21:1). We see a vision of life where "God Himself will be among them, and He will wipe away every tear from their eyes; and there will no longer be any death; there will no longer be any mourning, or crying, or pain;..." (21:3-4).

A new body will be ours as well. This body will never hurt; it will never decay; it will never need a hip replacement; or will it ever die. Your new heavenly bodies will last forever. Your soul and your spirit will possess a "heaven suit" that will not perish, allowing you to live forever with the Lord.

> *For to me, to live is Christ and to die is gain.*
> *But if I am to live on in the flesh, this will mean*
> *fruitful labor for me; and I do not know which to choose.*
> *But I am hard-pressed from both directions, having the*
> *desire to depart and be with Christ, for that is very much better;*
> *yet to remain on in the flesh is more necessary for your sake.*
> PHILIPPIANS 1:21-24

Between Now and Then

> *And this is eternal life, that they may know Thee,*
> *the only true God, and Jesus Christ whom Thou hast sent.*
> JOHN 17:3-4

> **Eternal life with Christ begins as soon as we receive Christ into our lives and experience the spiritual birth.**

For the rest of our earthly existence, our bodies will be confined to the limitations of time and the physical world. *But not so with our spirits.* Eternal life with Christ begins as soon as we receive Christ into our lives and experience the spiritual birth. We are now the adopted sons and daughters of the living God and we have an *eternal* inheritance that is ours *now.* Every minute of our day here on earth should be seen through *eternal eyes.*

> *Therefore we do not lose heart, but though our outer*
> *man is decaying, yet our inner man is being renewed day by day.*
> *For momentary, light affliction is producing for us an eternal weight*
> *of glory far beyond all comparison, while we look not at the things*
> *which are seen, but at the things which are not seen; for the things which*
> *are seen are temporal, but the things which are not seen are eternal.*

2 CORINTHIANS 4:16-18

As our bodies head toward the grave and our souls and spirits head toward heaven, our true focus needs to be on the *"inner* man." Certainly, we will continually face the limitations and decay of the *"outer* man." The reality and struggles of illness and pain are not to be minimized but they are to be put in perspective. And the biblical perspective is that these afflictions are momentary and light *compared* to the eternal glory that awaits...a glory that cannot be comprehended in this time-space dimension. That's why we are to focus on the inner spiritual man. It's the part of us that is being renewed day by day, conforming us to Christ, and allowing us to experience eternal life with Him *now.*

> **As our bodies head toward the grave and our souls and spirits head toward heaven, our true focus needs to be on the *"inner* man."**

Vision is not to be locked on the things that will not last, but on those things that will last forever.

> *If then you have been raised up with Christ, keep seeking*
> *the things above, where Christ is, seated at the right hand of God.*
> *Set your mind on the things of God, for you have died,*
> *and your life is hidden with Christ in God.*
> COLOSSIANS 2:8-9

In the midst of this temporal world our eyes are to be focused on the things of eternity. As hardship, stress, and difficulty swirl around us, God and the things of God are to be at the forefront of our thought. Through eternal eyes, we can see that we are not of this world, but are truly part of the kingdom of heaven. Pastor Jan Hettinga states it this way in his book, Follow Me:

Jesus' mission on earth was to provide access to the kingdom of God for all who would repent of their insurrection and revolt against the Creator. He did this by substituting Himself as the lightning rod for God's righteous indignation and justice. Without question, God's offer of reentry into the realm of His eternal kingdom is only available through the work on the cross.

Yet Jesus did not call the cross or His death and resurrection the good news. For Jesus, the kingdom was the good

news. *The magnificent work of the cross is the beginning.*
Atonement, reconciliation, redemption, justification, and pro-
pitiation are all essential ingredients of the gospel, but the
theme of the good news is the rest, freedom, peace, and high
investment value of living life under the leadership of the
Sovereign Lord of heaven and earth.

(emphasis mine)

When we look at ourselves and at our world with eternal eyes, the complete victory that Christ won comes into view. From this vantage point, eternal eyes gives us a powerful perspective for everyday living in His kingdom, and a supernatural peace as we look to the future. We are able to surrender our will to the loving and caring King of kings and Lord of Lords.

Seeing Life through Eternal Eyes

So teach us to number our days,
that we may present to You a heart of wisdom.
PSALM 90:12

We were created to recognize our mortality, and then focus our passions, hopes, and resources on something greater. It's one of the great mysteries of the faith that *real* life was never about *this* life in the first place. Jesus said, "*I* am the way, and the truth, and the *life*" (John 14:6). Christ brought everything there is into being (John 1:3), and He will be the one who will be at the center of the stage when eternity becomes the only reality (Revelation 22). In between, here and now, God designed us for a life that supersedes all we can see, a life that outlasts anything material. We have already entered His kingdom and eternity as He calls us to see life with eyes that aren't focused on what is temporary, but are fixed on the things that will never end.

Eternal eyes allow us to see the *truth in perspective.* As we do, a remarkable, moment-by-moment transformation begins to take place. When we align our minds and our hearts with His will and what is objectively true about this earthly life and physical death, our vision is propelled toward the things that will last forever. But how we need to pray for faith and wisdom! Our finite brains are wholly incapable of grasping even the minutest sliver of what eternity is. But we *must* see it! Only then can all of earthly life and everything it contains be measured properly. Only by capturing a glimpse of forever can we compare the insignificance of the things around us to the significance of the things that await us.

Eternal eyes allow us to set our minds on the things above and actually free us to rest in the Lord—not just because of the peace and health that it brings us now, but because it prepares us for the everlasting intimacy that will finally be fully realized in heaven. That intimacy can be *tasted* in continual fellowship and service with Him right now, but a great *feast* awaits us on the other side of the grave. Our final union with Him will be like the great ticker tape parade for the veteran who has come home after a long and bitter war. It will be like the elaborate wedding celebration after the intense expectation of engagement. It will be our Lord with us, in uninterrupted, unhindered, unadulterated intimacy and union.

> **This is one of the great rewards of living by design: to take eternal principles and begin to apply them *now*— so that the feast, the parade, and the celebration might begin *now*.**

This is one of the great rewards of living by design: to take eternal principles and begin to apply them *now*—so that the feast, the parade, and the celebration might begin *now*. That's why we want to break the cycle of self-effort and begin abiding in Christ and walking in the Spirit. When we get the focus of life off ourselves and onto Him, we can be with Him in real ways.

Eternal eyes will also allow us to see the true value of the things around us and prompt us to adjust our priorities accordingly. That's important, because in most cases, we've got it absolutely backward. Homes, bank accounts, clothes, body image, health, 401Ks, and cars...none of these things will last. Yet don't we cling to them in desperation, as if they were the most valuable of all things? How about our reputations and our work? Don't we panic when these things are threatened, as if our very lives depended upon them? Eternal eyes show us that these things are passing away as well. It's only a matter of time until they too fade completely from memory. In place of these things that have no lasting value, eternal eyes allow us to begin to focus on the souls of others, one of the few things that will last.

> "Do not lay up for yourselves treasures upon earth,
> where moth and rust destroy, and where thieves break in and steal.
> But lay up for yourselves treasures in heaven, where neither moth
> nor rust destroys, and where thieves do not break in or steal;
> for where your treasure is, there will your heart be also."...

*But seek first His kingdom and His righteousness;
and all these things shall be added to you. Therefore do not
be anxious for tomorrow; for tomorrow will care for itself.
Each day has enough trouble of its own.*
MATTHEW 6:19-21, 34

> Seeing everything
> from the vantage
> point of eternity
> gives us a clear
> view of what has
> true value and what
> doesn't. As we begin
> to have an eternal
> perspective, focus
> on self begins to
> fade and we
> become concerned
> about others.

Seeing everything from the vantage point of eternity gives us a clear view of what has true value and what doesn't. As we begin to have an eternal perspective, focus on self begins to fade and we become concerned about others. Material possessions begin to fade and our relationship with others and our God comes to the forefront. The sweet aroma of God's love begins to flow to others around us. In his book, *Ruthless Trust,* Brennan Manning elaborates on the change this new perspective brings:

In our turning toward God we are learning to turn away from "the world, the flesh, and the Devil." We are also turning away from ourselves as the be-all and end-all of life, for we are slowly but surely realizing that God is truly the heart and center of all things.

If anyone wishes to come after Me, he must deny himself, and take up his cross and follow Me. For whoever wishes to save his life shall lose it; but whoever loses his life for My sake and the gospel's shall save it. For what does it profit a man to gain the whole world, and forfeit his soul? For what shall a man give in exchange for his soul?
MARK 8:34-37

Three things and three things only will outlast time: God, the souls and spirits of humans, and the Word of God. The person who sees life with the eternal eyes of wisdom will invest in these three above all else. That's why Paul said, "I consider all things loss in view of the surpassing value of knowing Christ Jesus my Lord, for whom I have suffered the loss of all things, and count them but rubbish so that I might gain Christ..." (Philippians 3:8). That's why we are called to, "Go therefore and make disciples of all nations..." (Matthew 28:19). That's why we are to aim our lives toward eternity...toward that day in heaven when souls from every tribe and nation will join together to worship the Lamb (Revelation 7:9-10). The significance of being involved in such a process is unfathomable: By choice, the temporary and fleeting moments that make up earthly life can be invested in the kingdom of heaven that has no end!

Lift your eyes to the sky, then look to the earth beneath;
For the sky will vanish like smoke, and the earth
will wear out like a garment and its inhabitants
will die in like manner. But My salvation will be forever,
and My righteousness will not wane."

ISAIAH 51:6

> By choice, the temporary and fleeting moments that make up earthly life can be invested in the kingdom of heaven that has no end!

Eternal eyes will allow you to see each day for what it is: A passing moment in time that cannot be preserved, but only experienced. The "glory days" of the past are history, nothing more. Ecclesiastes 7:10 challenges us by saying, "Do not say, 'Why is it that the former days were better than these?' For it is not from wisdom that you ask about this." Neither should we be concerned about the future. "So do not worry about tomorrow; for tomorrow will care for itself" (Matthew 6:34). We are called to live each day, each moment, one by one. The present is all you have! You can't live in the past and the future never comes. God is feeding you life one little bite at a time. You can choose to savor every morsel...or you can wish them away with futile thoughts about what will never be.

As you begin to look with eternal eyes, your soul will be drawn to the unavoidable conclusion that your temporary physical life on this earth has a purpose that extends into the never ending future. Ponder the fact that you've been created for a *current* purpose that will *outlive* your earthly existence. If you find that purpose, your life on earth will finally have meaning, direction, and vision. How will that direction change your life on a moment-by-moment basis? How might that vision change the entire course of your life? God Himself only knows. But guided by your eternal eyes, He will show you how He wants to live His life through you. He will show you how together He intends to touch human souls with the expression of His Word in a way that brings glory to Him.

> We are called to live each day, each moment, one by one. The present is all you have! You can't live in the past and the future never comes.

Yes, eternal eyes are essential to resting in the Lord and setting your mind on Him. Consequently, eternal eyes will pull your life into action, igniting a passion for what is on the very heart of God. As you begin to see as He sees, His Spirit will stimulate your mind, aligning your desires with His will. Moment-by-moment you will allow Him to use your body as His instrument and mouthpiece of love, under the power of His grace working through you.

Let us also lay aside every encumbrance and the sin
which so easily entangles us, and let us run with endurance
the race that is set before us, fixing our eyes on Jesus,
the author and perfecter of faith...
HEBREWS 12:1-2

Home at Last

For now we see in a mirror dimly, but then face to face;
now I know in part, but then I will know fully just as I
also have been fully known. But now faith, hope, love,
abide these three; but the greatest of these is love.
1 CORINTHIANS 13:12-13

This world is not our home; we are just "passing through." As the familiar song proclaims, "Soon and very soon, we are going to see the King." On that amazing day, we will step out of our fleshly earth suit, leave time behind, and be free from all the lies, doubt, disease, and pain that have been our constant companions. We will leave behind the hardship, the stress, and the anger. With all these things we are much too familiar. But what we are headed for is wondrous beyond our greatest imagination.

Even the sharpest of eternal eyes cannot fully fathom what lies ahead. In that day, we will know Him as He knows us now. Our pride, arrogance, and deceit will evaporate in the complete understanding of who He is. Manipulation and greed will dissolve as His pure, unadulterated love engulfs us in inexhaustible quantity. Contemporary musician Bart Millard tried to capture the wonder of what lies ahead in his song, "I Can Only Imagine:"

I can only imagine,
What it will be like, when I walk by Your side.
Surrounded by Your glory, what will my heart feel?
Will I dance for You Jesus, or in awe of You be still?
Will I stand in Your presence, or to my knees will I fall?
Will I sing Hallelujah; will I be able to speak at all?
I can only imagine.
I can only imagine.

In those words we find a summary of our great hope. Our afflictions, as terminal as they might seem, are only momentary. And death, the most feared of all realities, will prove to be only a gateway into a glory that has no earthly comparison; a glory that is not bound by time and it will saturate us in the very presence of the God Himself.

That's the way He designed life. May He grant us the grace and mercy to live by it.

Thanks be to God, who gives us the victory through
our Lord Jesus Christ. Therefore, my beloved brethren,
be steadfast, immovable, always abounding in the work of the Lord,
knowing that your toil is not in vain in the Lord.
1 CORINTHIANS 15:57-58.

Now may the God of peace Himself sanctify you entirely;
and may your spirit and soul, and body be preserved complete,
without blame at the coming of our Lord Jesus Christ.
Faithful is He who calls you, and He also will bring it to pass.
2 THESSALONIANS 5:23-24

References

CHAPTER 2 Stress

Cooper, K, "Antioxidant Revolution", 94-10134 CIP, Thomas Nelson Publishing 1994.

Das, U. "Obesity, Metabolic Syndrome X, and Inflammation." *Nutrition* 18. (2001): 430-432.

Davies, Calvin. "Oxidative stress: The paradox of aerobic life." Biochem Soc Symp 61 (1995): 1-31

Davies K, "Oxidative Stress, Antioxidant Defenses, and Damage Removal, Repair and Replacement Systems." Life, 50:279-289 2000.

Knight JA. "Diseases related to oxygen-derived free radicals." Ann clin Lab Sci 1995 mar-Apr;25(2):111-21.

Landsberg, Lewis, et al. "Physiology and Pharmacology of the Autonomic Nervous System." Harrison's Principles of Internal Medicine 14th Edition [McGraw-Hill] 430-444

Lefer, David, "Oxidative Stress and Cardiac Disease." Am J Med. 2000;109:315-323

Mccord Joe, "The Evolution of Free Radical and Oxidative Stress." Am J Med 2000;108:652-659.

Moller P., H. Wallin, and L. Knudsen. "Oxidative stress associated with exercise, psychological stress, and life-style factors." Chemico-Biological Interactions 102 (1996): 17-36.

Ross, R., "Atherosclerosis-an Inflammatory Disease." *New England Journal of Medicine* 340, (1999): 115-123.

S. J. Stohs. "The role of free radicals in toxicity and disease." Journal of Basic and Clinical Physiology and Pharmacology 6 (1995): 3-4, 205-228.

20th U. S. Public Health Services Report released in 1986 by C. Everet Koop, M. D.

Young IS, "Antioxidants in health and disease." J Clin Pathol 2001 Mar;54(3):176-86.

CHAPTER 7 Exercise

Bjorntorp, P., et al. "The Effect of Physical Training on Insulin Production in Obesity." *Metabolism* 19. (1970): 631-638.

Helmrich, S.P., et al. "Physical Activity and Reduced Occurrence of Non-Insulin Dependent Diabetes Mellitus." *New England Journal of Medicine* 325. (1991): 147-152.

Holloszy, J.O., et.al. "Effects of Exercise on Glucose Tolerance and Insulin Resistance." *Acta Medica Scandinavica* 711. (1996): 55-65.

Hu, FB, et al. "Television Watching and Other Sedentary Behaviors in Relation to Risk of Obesity and Type 2 Diabetes Mellitus in Women." *JAMA* 289, (2003): 1785-1791.

Koivisto, V., and R.A. DeFronzo. "Physical Training and Insulin Sensitivity." *Diabetes Metabolism Reviews* 1. (1986): 445-481.

Leon, A.S., et al. "Effects of Vigorous Walking Program on Body Composition, and Carbohydrate and Lipid Metabolism of Obese Young Men." *Journal of Clinical Nutrition* 33 (1979):1776-1787.

Mayer-Davis, E.J., et al. "Intensity and Amount of Physical Activity in Relation to Insulin Sensitivity." *JAMA* 279. (1998): 669-674

20th U. S. Public Health Services Report released in 1986 by C. Everet Koop, M. D.

Yamanouchi, K.T., et al. "Daily Walking Combined with Diet Therapy is Useful Means for Obese NIDDM Patients Not Only to Reduce Body Weight But Also to Improve Insulin Sensitivity." *Diabetes Care* 18. (1995): 775-778.

CHAPTER 8 Healthy Diet

Allred, J.B. "Too Much of a Good Thing? An Overemphasis on Eating Low-Fat Foods May be Contributing to the Alarming Increase in Overweight Among US Adults." *Journal of the American Diet Association* 95. (1995): 417-418.

American Diabetes Association. "Type 2 Diabetes in Children and Adolescents." *Diabetes Care* 22. (2000): 381-389.

Bantle, J.P., et al. "Postprandial Glucose and Insulin Responses to Meals Containing Different Carbohydrates in Normal and Diabetic Subjects." *New England Journal of Medicine* 309. (1983): 7-12.

Bjorntorp, P., et al. "The Glucose Uptake of Human Adipose Tissue in Obesity." *European Journal of Clinical Investigation* 1. (1971): 480-485.

Blanco, I., and S.B. Roberts. "High Glycemic Index Foods, Over-Eating, and Obesity." *Pediatrics* 103. (1999): E261-E266.

Block G. "Dietary guidelines and the results of food surveys." *American Journal of Clinical Nutrition* 53 (1991): 3565-75

Brand, J.C., et al. "The Glycemic Index is Easy and Works in Practice." *Diabetes Care* 20. (1997): 1628-1629.

Ceriello, A., et al. "Meal Induced Oxidative Stress and Low-Density Lipoprotein Oxidation in Diabetes: The Possible Role of Hyperglycemia." *Metabolism* 48. (1999): 1503-1508.

Ceriello, A., and M. Pirisi. "Is Oxidative Stress the Missing Link Between Insulin Resistance and Atherosclerosis?" (letter). *Diabetologia* 38. (1995): 1484-1485.

Colgan, Michael. *The New Nutrition.* Apple Publishing, (1995).

Das, U. "Obesity, Metabolic Syndrome X, and Inflammation." Nutrition 18. (2001): 430-432.

Evans, D.J., et al. "Relationship Between Skeletal Muscle Insulin Resistance, Insulin-Mediated Glucose Disposal, and Insulin Binding: Effects of Obesity and Body Fat Topography." *Journal of Clinical Investigation* 74. (1984): 1515-1525.

Flegal, K.M., et al. "Overweight and Obesity in the US: Prevalence and Trends, 1960-1994." *International Journal of Obesity* 22. (1998): 39-47.

Fontaine, K.R., et al. "Years of Life Lost Due to Obesity." *JAMA* 289. (2003): 187-193.

Ford, E.S., et al. "Prevalence of the Metabolic Syndrome Among US Adults." *JAMA* 287 (2002): 356-359.

Foster-Powell, K., and J.B. Miller. "International Tables of Glycemic Index." *American Journal of Clinical Nutrition* 62. (1995): 871S-890S.

Foster-Powell, K., Brand-Miller, J.C, and Holt, S.H.A. "International Table of Glycemic Index and Glycemic Load Values: 2002." *American Journal of Clinical Nutrition* 76, (2002): 5-56.

Holt, S., et al "Relationship of Satiety to Postprandial Glycaemic, Insulin and Cholecystokinin Responses." *Appetite* 18. (1992): 129-141.

Jenkins, D., et al. "Glycemic Index of Foods: A Physiological Basis for Carbohydrate Exchange." *American Journal of Clinical Nutrition* 34. (1981): 362-366.

Jenkins, D., et al. "Nibbling Versus, Gorging: Metabolic Advantages of Increased Meal Frequency." *New England Journal of Medicine* 321. (1989): 929-934.

Lawrence, M., et al. "Oral Glucose Loading Acutely Attenuates Endothelium-Dependent Vasodilation in Healthy Adults Without Diabetes: An Effect Prevented by Vitamins C and E. Journal of the American College of Cardiology 36. (2000): 2185-2191.

Leathwood, P., Pollet, P. "Effects of Slow Release Carbohydrates in the Form of Bean Flakes on the Evolution of Hunger and Satiety in Man." *Appetite* 10. (1988): 1-11.

Ludwig, D.S., et al. "High Glycemic Index Foods, Overeating, and Obesity." *Pediatrics* 103. (1999): e26.

Ludwig, D.S. "The Glycemic Index: Physiological Mechanisms Relating to Obesity, Diabetes, and Cardiovascular Disease." *JAMA* 287. (2002): 2412-2423.

Martin-Moreno, J., et al. "Dietary Fat, Olive Oil Intake and Breast Cancer Risk." *International Journal of Cancer* 58. (1994): 774-780.

Munoz KA, et al. "Food intake of United States children and adolescents compared with recommendations." Pediatrics 100: No. 3 (September 1997): 323-329

Nuttall, F.Q., et al. "Effect of Protein Ingestion on the Glucose and Insulin Response to a Standardized Oral Glucose Load." *Diabetes Care* 7. (1984): 465-70.

Pinkey, J.A., et al. "Endothelial Cell Dysfunction: Cause of the Insulin Resistance Syndrome." *Diabetes* 46. (1997): S9-S13.

Reaven, G.M. "Syndrome X: 6 Years Later." *Journal of Internal Medicine Suppl* 736. (1994): 13-22.

Rossetti, L., et al. "Glucose Toxicity." *Diabetes Care* 13. (1990): 610-630.

Schlosser, Eric. *Fast Food Nation,* Mifflin Company, (2002).

Subar, A.F., et al. "Dietary Sources of Nutrients Among US Children, 1989-1991." *Pediatrics* 102. (1998): 913-923.

Torjesen, P.A., et al. "Lifestyle Changes May Reverse Development of the Insulin Resistance Syndrome." *Diabetes Care* 30. (1997): 26-31.

Troiano, R.P., et al. "Overweight Prevalence and Trends for Children and Adolescents: The National Health and Nutrition Examination Surveys, 1963-1991." *Arch Pediatric. Adolesc. Med.* 149. (1995): 1085-1091.

Visioli, F., and C. Galli. "Olive Oil Phenols and Their Potential Effects on Human Health." *Journal of Agnc. Food Chem.* 46. (1998): 42922-4296.

Weil, Andrew, *Eating Well for Optimal Health.* Alfred A. Knopf (2000)

Willett, W., et al. "Mediterranean Diet Pyramid: A Cultural Model for Healthy Eating." *American Journal of Clinical Nutrition* 61. (1995): 1402S-1406S.

Wolever, T., et al. "The Glycemic Index: Methodology and Clinical Implications." *American Journal of Clinical Nutrition* 54. (1991): 846-854.

Wood, Christine, *How to Get Kids to Eat Great & Love It!* Griffin Publishing; 2nd edition, (2001).

CHAPTER 9 Optimizing God's Defenses: Nutritional Supplementation

Block G, "Dietary guidelines and the results of food surveys." *American Journal of Clinical Nutrition* 53 (1991): 3565-75

Davies, Calvin. "Oxidative stress: The paradox of aerobic life." Biochem Soc Symp 61 (1995): 1-31

Davies K, "Oxidative Stress, Antioxidant Defenses, and Damage Removal, Repair and Replacement Systems." Life, 50:279-289 2000.

Garewal HS. Chemoprevntion of Cancer. Hematol Oncol Clin North Am 1991 Feb, 5(1):69-77.

Singh V, "Premalignant Lesions Role of Antioxidant vitamins and B Carotene is risk reduction and prevention of malignant transformation." AM J Clin Nutr 1991;53:386S-90S.

Griendling, K.K., et al. "Oxidative Stress and Cardiovascular Disease." *Circulation* 96. (1997): 3264-3265

Jha, P., et al. "The Antioxidant Vitamins and Cardiovascular Disease. A Critical Review of Epidemilogic and Clinical Trial Data." *Annals of Internal Medicine* 123. (1995): 860-872.

Knight JA. "Diseases related to oxygen-derived free radicals." Ann clin Lab Sci 1995 mar-Apr;25(2):111-21.

Kovacic P, "Mechanisms of Carcinogenesis: Focus on Oxidative Stress," Current Med. Chemistry 2001; Vol. 8, No. 7; 773-796

Langsjoen H., P. Langsjoen, et al. "Usefulness of Coenzyme Q10 in clinical cardiology: A long-term study." Molecular Aspects of Medicine 15 (1994 [supplement]): S165-S175.

Lefer, David, "Oxidative Stress and Cardiac Disease." Am J Med. 2000;109:315-323

Mccord Joe, "The Evolution of Free Radical and Oxidative Stress." Am J Med 2000;108:652-659.

Moller, P., H. Wallin, and L. Knudsen. "Oxidative stress associated with exercise, psychological stress, and life-style factors." Chemico-Biological Interactions 102 (1996): 17-36.

Ross, R., "Atherosclerosis-an Inflammatory Disease." *New England Journal of Medicine* 340, (1999): 115-123.

Steinberg, D., "Antioxidants in the prevention of human atherosclerosis." Summary of the proceedings of a National Heart, Lung, and Blood Institute workshop: September 5-6. 1991.

Stohs, S. J.. "The role of free radicals in toxicity and disease." Journal of Basic and Clinical Physiology and Pharmacology 6 (1995): 3-4, 205-228.

Strand, Ray. *What Your Doctor Doesn't Know About Nutritional Medicine May Be Killing You.* Thomas Nelson Publishers. (2002).

Thompson, K.H., and D.V. Godlin. "Micronutrients and Antioxidants in the Progression of Diabetes." *Nutrition Reseatrch* 15. (1995): 1377-1410.

Young IS, "Antioxidants in health and disease." J Clin Pathol 2001 Mar;54(3):176-86.

Recommended Food List

Listed in this section are the recommended foods you need to consider when making your meal and snack choices. These are broken down into three categories: Desirable, Moderately Desirable, and Least Desirable. Perfection is not the goal, but rather, 75 to 80 percent of your food choices should be coming from the desirable food recommendations and 20 to 25 percent from the moderately desirable food recommendations. No more than 5 percent of your food choices should ever come from the least desirable food recommendations.

The carbohydrates are listed with their respective glycemic index and glycemic load. Several considerations were made before placing a particular food into its specific category such as: quality of nutrients contained, glycemic index, glycemic load, and whether it contains good proteins and fats.

DESIRABLE CARBOHYDRATES

	GLYCEMIC INDEX	GLYCEMIC LOAD
Fruits		
Apple	38	6
Apricots	57	5
Cherries	22	3
Grapefruit	25	3
Grapes	43	7
Kiwi Fruit	47	5
Mango	47	5
Orange	42	5
Peach	28	4
Peach (canned in natural juice)	38	4
Pear	38	4
Pear (canned in natural juice)	43	5
Pineapple	59	7
Plums	24	7
Watermelon	72	4
Vegetables		
Artichokes	[0]	0
Avocado	[0]	0
Beet	64	5
Broccoli	[0]	0
Cabbage	[0]	0
Carrots	47	3
Cauliflower	[0]	0
Celery	[0]	0
Cucumber	[0]	0
Peas	48	3
Leafy Vegetables (spinach, lettuce)	[0]	0
Squash	[0]	0
Yam	37	13

DESIRABLE CARBOHYDRATES

	GLYCEMIC INDEX	GLYCEMIC LOAD
Legumes		
Beans, butter	31	7
Beans, kidney	28	7
Beans, black	20	5
Chickpeas		
(garbanzo beans, Bengal gram)	28	8
Lentils	29	5
Lentils, green, dried	30	5
Lentils, red	26	5
Soy Beans	18	1
Breads		
Coarse Barley Kernel Bread:		
75% Kernels	27	7
80% Kernels		
(20% white flour)	34	8
Oat Bran Bread	47	9
Rye Kernel Bread		
(pumpernickel)	41	5
Sourdough Rye	53	6
Healthy Choice Wheat Bread		
(Con Agra Inc., USA)	55	8
Soy and Linseed Bread		
(packet mix in bread oven)		
(Con Agra Inc., USA)	50	5
Silver Hills Sprouted Bread	Has not been tested	
Ezekiel Sprouted Bread	Has not been tested	

DESIRABLE CARBOHYDRATES

	GLYCEMIC INDEX	GLYCEMIC LOAD
Breakfast Cereals		
All-Bran (Kellogg's, USA)	38	9
Bran Buds (Kellogg's, Canada)	58	7
Bran Buds with Psyllium (Kellogg's, Canada)	47	6
Hot Cereal, Apple and Cinn. (Con Agra Inc., USA)	37	8
Hot Cereal, unflavored (Con Agra Inc., USA)	25	13
Oat Bran, raw	55	3
Cereal Grains		
Barley, pearled	25	11
Rice, parboiled (Uncle Ben's)	38	14
Rice, parboiled, long grain (Canada)	38	14
Rye	34	13
Wheat, whole kernels	41	14
Wheat, cracked (bulgur)	48	12
Dairy Products		
Yogurt, low fat	31	9
Soy Milk	44	8
Milk, skim	32	4

DESIRABLE CARBOHYDRATES

	GLYCEMIC INDEX	GLYCEMIC LOAD
Nuts		
Almonds	[0]	0
Cashew Nuts	22	3
Hazelnuts	[0]	0
Macadamia	[0]	0
Pecan	[0]	0
Peanuts	14	1
Walnuts	[0]	0
Sugars and Sweeteners		
Fructose (Granulated)	19	2
Stevia	0	0

MODERATELY DESIRABLE CARBOHYDRATES

	GLYCEMIC INDEX	GLYCEMIC LOAD
Fruits		
Apple Juice, unsweetened	40	10
Apricots, canned in light syrup	64	12
Banana	52	12
Orange Juice	52	12
Peach, canned in heavy syrup	58	9
Prunes	29	10
Strawberries	40	10
Vegetables		
Corn, sweet	54	9
Pumpkin	75	3
Rutabaga	72	7

MODERATELY DESIRABLE CARBOHYDRATES

	GLYCEMIC INDEX	GLYCEMIC LOAD
Potato		
New Potato	62	13
Sweet Potato	61	17
Legumes		
Beans, baked	48	7
Beans, dried	29	9
Beans, black-eyed	42	13
Beans, navy	38	12
Beans, lima	32	10
Pinto Beans	39	10
Bread		
Barley Flour Breads	67	9
Whole-Wheat Barley Flour Bread with Sourdough (lactic acid)	53	10
Whole-Wheat Rye Bread	58	8
Coarse Wheat Kernel Bread, (80% intact kernels)	52	12
Breakfast Cereals		
All-Bran (Kellogg's, Canada)	50	9
Cream of Wheat	66	17
Oatmeal, rolled oats	58	13
Cereal Grains		
Barley, cracked	66	21
Buckwheat (Canada)	54	16
Cornmeal, boiled in salt water (Canada)	68	9
Sweet Corn (USA)	60	20
Taco Shells, cornmeal-based	68	8
Couscous, boiled	65	23
Rice, long grain, wild (Uncle Ben's)	54	20

MODERATELY DESIRABLE CARBOHYDRATES

	GLYCEMIC INDEX	GLYCEMIC LOAD
Cereal Grains cont.		
Rice, basmati, boiled	58	22
Rice, brown	55	18
Rice, par boiled (USA)	72	18
Bakery Goods		
Banana Cake, made without sugar	55	16
Chocolate Cake		
(Betty Crocker)	38	20
Muffin, apple without sugar	48	9
Cookies		
Digestives (Canada)	59	10
Oatmeal (Canada)	54	9
Pasta and Noodles		
Fettuccine, egg	40	18
Linguine	52	23
Macaroni	47	23
Noodles, instant	47	19
Spaghetti, white	44	21
Spaghetti, whole wheat	37	16
Sugars and Sweeteners		
Honey	55	10

LEAST DESIRABLE CARBOHYDRATES

	GLYCEMIC INDEX	GLYCEMIC LOAD
Bakery Goods		
Angel Food Cake	67	19
Croissant	67	17
Doughnut, cake	76	17
Muffin, oat, raisin	54	14
Muffin, banana	65	16
Muffin, bran	60	15
Pound Cake (Sara Lee)	54	15
Cookies		
Graham Wafers		
(Christie Brown, Canada)	74	14
Vanilla Wafers (Canada)	77	14
Dairy Products		
Ice Cream	61	8
Ice Cream, low fat	47	5
Ice Cream, premium	37	4
Milk	27	3
Pudding	47	7
Yogurt	36	3
Fruits		
Raisins	64	28
Cranberry Juice Cocktail	68	24
Dates	50	12
Figs	61	16
Pineapple Juice	46	15
Vegetables		
Parsnips	97	12
Potato		
Baked, white	85	26
Instant, mashed	85	17
Mashed Potato	92	18

LEAST DESIRABLE CARBOHYDRATES

	GLYCEMIC INDEX	GLYCEMIC LOAD
Breads		
Bagel, white	72	25
Coarse Oat Kernel Bread, 80%intact oat kernels	65	12
Hamburger Bun	61	9
Kaiser Rolls	73	12
White Flour bread	70	10
Whole-Wheat Flour Bread	71	8
Breakfast Cereals		
Bran Chex	58	11
Bran Flakes	74	15
Cheerios	74	15
Coco Pops	77	15
Corn Chex	83	21
Corn Flakes (Kellogg's, USA)	92	24
Cream of Wheat, instant	74	22
Golden Grahams	71	18
Grapenuts (Kraft, USA)	75	13
Grapenuts Flakes (Post, Canada)	80	17
Instant Oatmeal	66	17
Life (Quaker Oats Co., Canada)	66	16
Muesli (Canada)	66	16
Puffed Wheat	67	13
Raisin Bran (Kellogg's, USA)	61	12
Rice Chex (Nabisco, Canada)	89	21
Rice Krispies (Kellogg's, Canada)	82	21
Shredded Wheat (Nabisco, Canada)	83	17
Special K (Kellogg's, USA)	69	14
Total (General Mills, Canada)	76	17

LEAST DESIRABLE CARBOHYDRATES

	GLYCEMIC INDEX	GLYCEMIC LOAD
Cereal Grains		
Millet, boiled (Canada)	71	25
Noodles, rice (Australia)	76	37
Rice, white	72	30
Rice, long grain	56	23
Rice, long grain, quick-cooking variety	68	25
Rice, Jasmine (Thailand)	109	46
Rice, instant white	87	36
Snacks and Candy		
Corn Chips	42	11
Fruit Roll Ups	99	24
Jelly Beans	78	22
Mars Bars	68	26
Popcorn	72	24
Potato Chips	54	11
Pretzels	83	16
Snickers Bar	68	23
Twix	44	17
Sugars and Sweeteners		
Glucose	100	10
Lactose	46	5
Maltose	105	11
Sucrose (table sugar)	61	6
Alternative Sweeteners		
Xylitol	8	1
Splenda	0	0
Aspartame	0	0

Desirable Protein/Fat

Salmon
Mackerel
Trout
Tuna (once weekly at the most)
Sardines
Almonds (raw)
Walnuts (raw)
Soybeans
Flaxseed
Flaxseed oil (cold pressed)
Herring
Olives
Virgin olive oil
Avocado
Pumpkin seeds

Eggs (range fed chickens)
Peas
Beans
Lentils
Soymilk
Tofu
Soy Burgers
Turkey (skinless)
Turkey bacon
Turkey burgers
Hummus
Buffalo meat
Wild game meat (deer, elk,
    pheasant, quail)

Moderately Desirable Protein/Fat

Cashews
Pistachios
Macadamias
Mayonnaise (natural, made from
    olive, soy, or canola oils)
Eggs (commercial)
Peanuts
Peanut oil
Peanut butter (natural)
Canola oil (expeller-pressed)
Safflower oil
Sunflower oil
Sesame oil
Corn oil
Soy oil
Walnut butter
Hazelnuts

Skim milk
Low-fat cottage cheese
Low-fat yogurt
Halibut
Lean hamburger (90% plus)
Beef (lean cuts)
Chicken (skinless is better)
Beef Tenderloin
Top Sirloin
Flounder
Sole
Cod
Orange roughy
Duck
Shrimp
Crab

Least Desirable Protein/Fat

Margarine

Vegetable Shortening

Fried Foods

Deep Fat Fried Foods

Cottonseed oil

Butter

Coconut oil

Palm Kernel oil

Palm oil

Any oil that is Partially
   Hydrogenated (read labels)

Milk

Cheese

Ice cream

Cream

Bacon

Sausage

Hot dogs

Lunch meat

Pork

Pepperoni

Salami

Spareribs, pork

Ground beef

Lamb

Liver, chicken

Brain

Heart

Beef roasts (chuck)

Oysters

Lobster

About the Authors

Ray D. Strand, M. D., graduated from the University of Colorado Medical School and finished his post-graduate training at Mercy Hospital in San Diego, California. He has been involved in an active private family practice for the past thirty years, and has focused his practice on nutritional medicine over the past ten years while lecturing internationally on the subject. He is also the author of the best-selling *What Your Doctor Doesn't Know About Nutritional Medicine, Death by Prescription,* and *Healthy for Life.* Dr. Strand lives on a horse ranch in South Dakota with his lovely wife, Elizabeth. They have three grown children, Donny, Nick, and Sarah.

To reach this author by internet:
www.drraystrand.com
or
www.healthyandleanforlife.com

by mail:
Health Concepts
P. O. Box 9226
Rapid City, SD 57709

About the Authors

Bill Ewing is the Founder and CEO of Christian Life Ministries. Over the past 25 years, CLM has been reaching out with cutting-edge biblical counseling to those who are hurting, disillusioned, and burned-out. An international conference speaker and trainer, Bill is also the co-founder of The International Association of Biblical Counselors (IABC) and is a Charter Member of the Association of Exchanged Life Ministries. He started out his career as a professional baseball player following an excellent college career where he set the all-time collegiate home run record while attending the University of Wyoming. Bill lives with his wife Nancy in Rapid City, South Dakota and has 3 grown children; Jesse, Nic, and Kyle.

To reach this author by phone:
605-341-5305

by mail:
Bill Ewing
Christian Life Ministries
1948 N Plaza Drive
Rapid City, SD 57702